Waistline Workou

Medical Disclaimer: The information in this book is intended as a general guide, and in no way should be seen as a substitute for your doctor's own advice. All care is taken to ensure the information is free from error or omissions. No responsibility, however, can be accepted by the author, editor, publisher, or any other person involved in the preparation of the material for loss occasioned to any person acting or refraining from action as a result of the published information. Before commencing any new health program, diet or exercise, always consult your doctor.

The Body Coach Series

Waistline Workout

New diet and exercise plan to trim and tone your waistline and increase your energy levels

Paul Collins

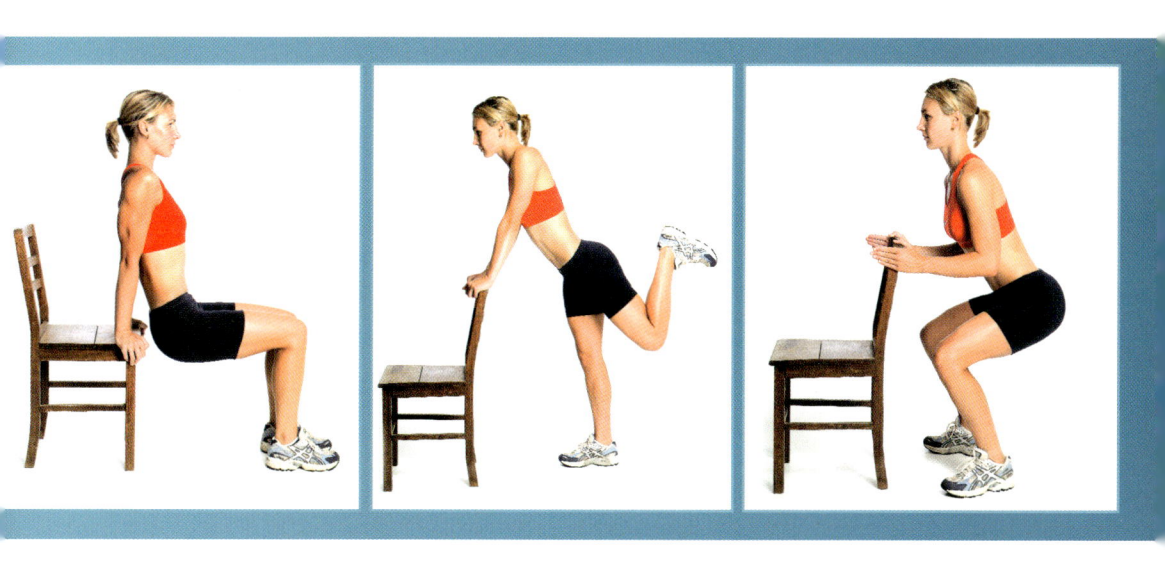

Meyer & Meyer Sport

British Library Cataloguing in Publication Data
A catalogue record for this book is available from the British Library

Paul Collins
Waistline Workout
Maidenhead: Meyer & Meyer Sport (UK) Ltd., 2010
ISBN 978-1-84126-285-7

All rights reserved, especially the right to copy and distribute, including the translation rights.
No part of this work may be reproduced – including by photocopy, microfilm or any other means – processed, stored electronically, copied or distributed in any form whatsoever without the written permission of the publisher.

© 2010 Paul Collins (text & photos)
and Meyer & Meyer Sport (UK) Ltd. (Layout)
Aachen, Adelaide, Auckland, Budapest, Cape Town, Graz, Indianapolis,
Maidenhead, Olten (CH), Singapore, Toronto
Member of the World
Sport Publishers' Association (WSPA)
www.w-s-p-a.org

Printed and bound by: B.O.S.S Druck und Medien GmbH, Germany
ISBN 978-1-84126-285-7
E-Mail: info@m-m-sports.com
www.m-m-sports.com

Contents

About the Author 6
A Word from the Body Coach® 7
Introduction 9
Waistline Workout Success Story 15

Step 1: Establishing a Healthy Eating Diet Plan 17
Recommended Dietary Intake (RDI) 19
RDI Vitamin and Mineral Diet Chart 21
RDI - Food Translation 24
Complex Carbohydrates 29
Proteins 32
Fat (Lipids) 35
Body Coach® Daily Food Portion Chart 36
Sample RDI Eating Day 38
Similar Energy, Different Size 40
Meal Choices 43

Step 2: Participating in Regular Daily Exercise 52
a. Body Audit 53
b. Exercise Plan 61
    Phase 1: Strength Training 63
    Phase 2: Heart and Lung Fitness 110
Becoming a WW Gold Medallist 113
Body Coach® 30-Minute WW Cardio Approach 113

Step 3: Successful Lifestyle Planning and Motivation .120
12-Week Action Plan 126
Monitoring Your Progress 130
WW Progress Summary Chart 132

Photo & Illustration Credits 136

Trademarks
Belly Busters®, Thigh Busters®, Body Coach®, The Body Coach®, 3 Hour Rule®, Spinal Unloading Block®, Posturefit®, Fastfeet®, Quickfeet®, BodyBell®, Coach Collins™, Australia's Personal Trainer™, Personal Training for Pets™, PT for Pets™, Speed for Sport™, 3B's Principle™, Waistline Workout™, Spin Box™ are all trademarks of Paul Collins.

About the Author

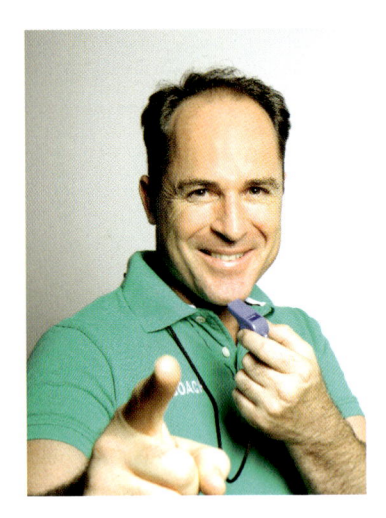

Paul Collins, Australia's Personal Trainer™, is founder of The Body Coach® fitness products, books, DVD's and educational coaching systems – helping people to get fit, lose weight, look good and feel great. Coaching since age 14, Paul has personally trained world-class athletes and teams in a variety of sports from track and field, squash, rugby, golf, soccer and tennis to members of the Australian World Championship Karate Team, Manly 1st Grade Rugby Union Team and members of the world-renowned Australian Olympic and Paralympic Swimming teams. Paul is an outstanding athlete in his own right, having played grade rugby league in the national competition, being an A-grade squash player, National Budokan Karate Champion and NSW State Masters Athletics Track & Field Champion.

A recipient of the prestigious 'Fitness Instructor of the Year Award' in Australia, Paul is regarded by his peers as the 'Trainers' Trainer' having educated thousands of fitness instructors and personal trainers and appeared on TV, radio and print media features. Over the past decade, Paul has presented to national sporting bodies including the Australian Track and Field Coaching Association, Australia Swimming Coaches and Teachers Association, Australian Rugby League, Australian Karate Federation and the Australian Fitness Industry as well as travelling to present a highly entertaining series of corporate health & well-being seminars for companies focused on a Body for Success™ in life and in business.

Paul holds a Bachelor of Physical Education degree from the Australian College of Physical Education. He is also a Certified Trainer and Assessor, Strength and Conditioning Coach with the Australian Sports Commission and Olympic Weight Lifting Club Power Coach with the Australian Weightlifting Federation. As a Certified Personal Trainer with Fitness Australia, Paul combines over two decades of experience as a talented athlete, coach and mentor for people of all age groups and ability levels in achieving their optimal potential.

In his free time, Paul enjoys competing in track and field, massage, travelling, nice food and movies. He resides in Sydney, Australia.

For more details visit: www.thebodycoach.com

A Word from the Body Coach®

Obesity levels are continually on the rise. The good news is that the *Waistline Workout* offers a total lifestyle solution in a manner that is easy to apply and brings with it long term results that matter. I've personally set out to provide you with practical solutions for you to achieve better health and a better body with my revolutionary Waistline Workout 3-Step Weight Loss System, based on:

Step 1: Establishing a Healthy Eating Diet Plan
Step 2: Participating in Regular Daily Exercise (including Body Audit)
Step 3: Successful Lifestyle Planning and Motivation – including a 12-Week Action Plan

The *Waistline Workout* is a simple, easy-to-follow roadmap to healthy eating, proper exercise and increasing your energy levels. Along the way, I provide you with a highly effective Lifestyle Planning System to help motivate and keep you on track whilst shedding those unwanted pounds (kilograms).

In Step 1 I'll show you a nutritionally balanced diet based on the recommended dietary intakes (RDI) required for maintaining good health. This includes categorizing these essential nutrients into the three major food groups commonly referred to as carbohydrate, protein and fat. To help gauge and monitor your progress, I have developed The Body Coach® Daily Food Portion Chart that makes dieting simple and easy to plan, implement and maintain, ensuring you gain all the essential nutrients required for good health all year round.

In Step 2 our first goal is a series of health benchmarks which allows you to establish goals, get the mind on task and make important lifestyle changes. These benchmarks are then re-tested throughout your 12-week journey to show you where improvements are occurring and keep your spirits high, because whilst one area may be unchanged another will be and you will see the gradual shift towards your overall success. Next, I guide you through a revolutionary two-tier training program to help improve your heart and lung (cardiovascular or aerobic) fitness as well as improving your strength and muscle tone. This unique training system has easy-to-follow exercise descriptions and illustrations as well as a weekly exercise planner that you can tick off each day as you perform each exercise, ensuring accountability to the Waistline Workout program.

In Step 3 you chart your progress, which helps you keep your eye on your goal. This is achieved through successful lifestyle planning and motivation strategies and a 12-Week action plan. By making a commitment to yourself and being accountable to the Waistline Workout at hand you will undergo a series of positive life changes and experiences towards achieving a fitter, slimmer and sexier body.

Waistline Workout teaches you the importance of focusing on the foods your body needs each day for good health as opposed to ones your body doesn't need or could go without. Most importantly, it shows you how to regain your body shape through a healthy eating plan and regular exercise that will change your outlook forever. So, not only will you lose weight off those hard to get at areas but you'll be better educated and positively satisfied.

Now, before you get started, one of most important statements to remember is that whilst you can't change the past – you can improve your future!

I look forward to working with you!

Paul Collins
The Body Coach®

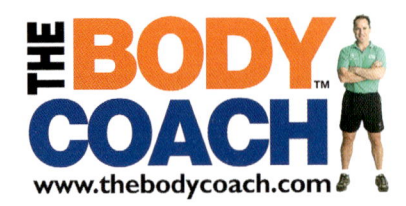

Introduction

Welcome to Waistline Workout (**WW**), the revolutionary 3-Step weight loss program for helping you to a slim, strong, healthy and sexier body. What separates **WW** from other weight loss programs is that here I show you *how* to get in shape, as opposed to just telling you *why*, in 3 easy steps – by showing you 'practically' what you need to do. This is because in most cases you already understand what is required and just need the guidance in how to put it all into practice.

WW excels because the recommendations here are based on scientific principles of healthy eating, regular exercise and lifestyle motivation. The good news is that I will guide you through a routine that will boost your body's ability to burn fat helping you drop inches off the hip, butt, thigh and waistline regions, whilst also shedding a few unwanted pounds (kilograms) of body fat weight that can have a substantial benefit on your total well-being.

As your Personal 'Body Coach®' my goal is simple: coaching you to achieve your best body shape ever – that's my promise to you! In order to do this, all I need is a commitment from you to stick with it, because I'm right here to guide you all the way.

With a positive approach you will be able to easily apply the WW plan into your own daily lifestyle. And, for those who may require a little extra guidance, I am available to you for coaching online at: www.thebodycoach.com.

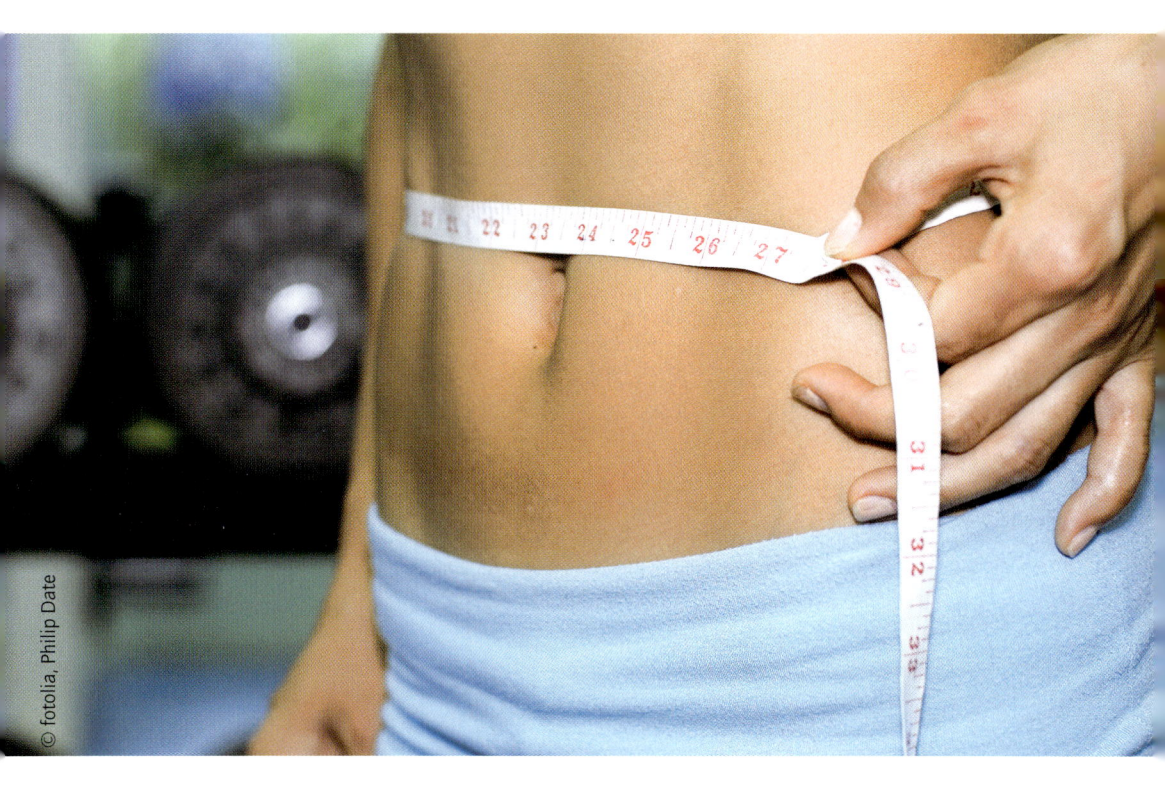

© fotolia, Philip Date

Bridging Science and Reality

Today, we are bombarded with too much information, more than we know what to do with. This deluge of information only makes it harder to apply ourselves to the facts that really matter when dealing with our health and well-being. As a result, WW has evolved from sorting through this endless array of nutritional research data and reported barriers to exercise and establishing a user-friendly weight loss program – based on scientific principles and techniques that are easy to adapt and can enhance one's lifestyle.

For this reason, don't be surprised by the simplicity of this program, as all the high tech scientific jargon has been summarized for you in a clear and uncomplicated format together with step-by-step coaching. So, whilst others are caught in the realm of confusion and always looking for solutions, you'll already be on the right pathway with the Waistline Workout 3-Step Weight Loss System.

Making the Necessary Changes

You'll be very surprised how a few simple changes in your life can make a major difference in the way you look and feel. By reading this book, I know you are ready for these changes to occur because you are becoming more conscious on the tasks at hand. Being conscious of where you are today in terms of your weight and how you got here should spark a need for change. By being conscious, you'll also become more interested, and you must have an interest before you have a belief. The more interested you become, the more you want to learn. With this in mind you'll begin to put the pieces of the puzzle together. It's not designed too happen overnight, but over time it will – and that's the exciting part. So, no matter what your age, you can feel excited and alive that WW will work for you in more ways than one – allowing you to grow and move forward in a youthful, positive way.

Body Fat Distribution

Body fat distribution is generally determined by genetics and gender. If you are male, your fat deposits are more likely to be around the belly, whilst females' fat is generally stored around the hip, butt and thigh region. The chemical characteristics of male belly fat from female thigh fat are quite different. The fat stored around the belly, whether in male or females, is more active than thigh fat meaning it circulates more readily throughout the blood stream. As a result, excess abdominal fat is seen to increase the risk of heart disease, diabetes, hypertension, various types of cancer and other health hazards. In order to reduce these risks the goal is trimming the waistline below 90cm for men and 80cm for women. Once this is achieved then reducing this even further is the next priority.

All forms of exercise are important in this instance, because when muscles are exercised the fat circulating around the blood stream can be utilized over time by the muscles. Whereas, if fat is released from emotional stress or overeating, the fat ends up clinging to the artery walls creating numerous health hazards. This is one of the reasons why diet and exercise is more successful than dieting alone in achieving a slimmer waistline.

Most people now realize the mistakes they have made in the past with dieting. Starving one's body or dieting alone generally leads to muscle of the upper body region being used as an energy source. It has also been observed that the area where you store fat first is also the area where you generally lose fat last. The resulting trimmer upper body and loss on the scales is dubbed by the now pear-shaped lower body that showcases the protruding hip, butt and thighs. As one of the most common questions from women, I have developed a unique balance between nutrition and exercise with WW that focuses on developing a more symmetrical body proportion. In essence, WW will show you how combining the Recommended Dietary Intake (RDI) of foods combined with muscle toning exercises for the upper body region and regular walking can help reduce the fat stored in the lower body region.

The Right Eating Plan

Good health is based on meeting specific nutritional needs. Diets that cut down on your food intake or limit specific foods in order to lose weight make it harder to meet your Recommended Dietary Intake (RDI). The RDI is the level of intake of essential nutrients considered, in the judgement of the National Health and Medical Research Council (NHMRC), to be adequate to meet the known nutritional needs of practically all healthy people. Specific RDIs are available for people in Australia, USA, England and Canada and are derived from estimates of requirements for each age/sex category and incorporate generous factors to accommodate variations in absorption and metabolism. Where I come into play is showing you how to combine this all together, because it's one thing telling you about it, and another showing how to do it – the major objective of WW.

People who are trying to lose weight can be at increased risk of deficiencies of a few key nutrients, particularly calcium, iron and zinc if they limit or cut down on specific foods. As a result, it is important to think about healthy foods that you need to include in your diet as part of the RDI as opposed to ones that only make you feel guilty. For optimal nutritional health, a varied diet providing adequate amounts of each essential nutrient from basic foods form the foundation of the WW Program.

The Recommended Dietary Intakes (RDI) are used with WW in three specific ways:

1. As an assessment of the adequacy of one's current eating plan
2. As a guide in planning diets and menus
3. As a guide to being better prepared and making better meal choices

Energy Intake versus Energy Output

With the escalation of high energy dense foods in one's diet over the past decade such as processed and manufactured foods, fast foods and sweets and a reduction in physical activity and movement levels, it seems the energy intake is overriding our energy output and the levels of obesity are increasing. You may recognize that when you overindulge in poor quality food and drink that you may feel emotionally flat. This is because physical, mental and emotional health are equally reliant on good nutrition.

Each day our body takes in fuel (or energy) as calories (or kilojoules) through the food we eat and the fluids we consume – except water which is calorie free. Our body needs a certain amount of energy and fluids each day for efficient functioning and survival. For this reason, if over an extended period of weeks, months or years, a person has consumed more energy than the body has used, it will get stored as fat – increasing one's body weight and waistline. Whereas on the other hand, if the energy intake is less than the energy output, the body may use some stored fat or muscle tissue as fuel and one's body weight may reduce over an extended period of time – as long as one's stress levels remain balanced.

The decision to turn this equation around ultimately comes from the decisions you make in terms of your food and lifestyle choices. As described previously, it is important to think about healthy foods that you need to include in your diet as part of the recommended dietary intake as opposed to what you shouldn't have because in most instances your current lifestyle and eating habits that are preventing you from losing weight.

Reducing the energy density of a meal and trading it with those as part of the RDI can help reverse this energy imbalance and regain the essential vitamins and minerals needed for good health and controlling your weight. Performing a self-assessment of your current eating habits over 7 days can remarkably help rebalance your life by helping you decipher the energy value of foods in order to make the right food choices. RDIs, Food Charts and other important aspects will be outlined in more detail in Step 1.

Food Relationships

Many relationships are formed with food and liquids over the years as a result of stress or a certain emotion or feeling of comfort that has eventually led to poor eating habits. The thing about these relationships is that they often go unnoticed and in many instances are not seen as a cause of poor health or increasing waistline because they have become a normal part of your everyday lifestyle and without them you feel lost. These relationships come in all forms and shapes and vary between individuals. But I assure you that you will have at least one or even more of these relationships that need to be recognized and accepted on your behalf that they are contributing to poor health and that you are the only person who can turn this around.

Each day we face multiple stress situations that lead to these food relationships. Take a look at the list on the following page to see what I mean. If any of these relate to you, it's important that you acknowledge them and make it a priority to turn them around. Just think of it like

INTRODUCTION

having your money in a bank account earning a low interest rate for too long. Now is the time to bring it to your attention, understand the reasons for change, attend to it by making it a priority to improve your lifestyle outlook, knowing that they will have to be reviewed on a regular basis – achieving greater results.

Here are a few examples to bring this to your attention. Tick any element that relates to you on a daily basis from the list below:

- [ ] I have regular cigarette or coffee breaks.
- [ ] I skip breakfast or only have a coffee first thing in the morning.
- [ ] I drink more than 4 cups of coffee a day.
- [ ] I consume either chocolate, chips, biscuits or sweets on a daily basis.
- [ ] I consume soft drinks.
- [ ] When I arrive home, I have a drink of alcohol or high energy treat.
- [ ] I drink alcohol every day often to calm myself down.
- [ ] I eat processed snacks or treats late into the evening.
- [ ] Fast food is my preferred choice for either breakfast, lunch or dinner.
- [ ] I eat the same meals every day such as the same breakfast, or lunch or dinner over and over again (often referred to as rut eating).
- [ ] I never stop and relax for either breakfast, lunch or dinner – always on the go.
- [ ] I don't drink any water, just other liquids.
- [ ] Any other similar occurrence: _____.

Now that I have brought these to your attention, from my experience it is a willingness to change these instances that will be the major turning point in your success. The relationship between feelings and a relationship with food (or drink) is becoming more understood. Key elements such as drinking more water as opposed to consuming alcohol, soft drinks, coffee, flavored drinks, etc., will ensure the pure water (around 1-3 liters a day) your body needs will be acquired and without the excess calories. Another example that can be used in breaking food relationships could be to change your habits when you arrive home from work, before eating, with exercise or active house duty or similar. By changing a habit and replacing it with a positive one, your health will be improved. If you need extra guidance with this, I recommend contacting a medical practitioner or psychologist.

Establishing Health Benchmarks

Health benchmarks such as the Body Mass Index (BMI), Waist Circumference, Healthy Weight Range, Blood Glucose, Blood Cholesterol and Blood Pressure Levels may all seem daunting in the beginning but they are necessary for helping you gauge where you stand today in terms of your size, weight, general health and your future well-being. The amazing thing is that measuring up to these recommended health ranges enables you to establish goals that are specific and measurable. Knowing where you stand today and where you need to be in the future is like having plans for building a house. WW provides you with the necessary materials and tools for completing your goal. How committed you are will tell you how long it will take to reach your goal. One major scientific fact about weight loss is guaranteed: Losing weight successfully is about striking the right balance between your diet, exercise (or movement) and lifestyle. With this approach you are reducing the risk of heart disease, osteoporosis, type 2 diabetes and many other health concerns. Establishing Health Benchmarks with the Body Audit will be outlined in more detail in Step 2.

Movement and Exercise

Scientific evidence clearly indicates that diet and exercise is the most effective approach for weight loss to occur. WW is a successful long term weight loss approach because it applies two key exercise elements as part of its overall program that focuses on developing more a symmetrical body proportion.

These two key exercise elements include:
1. Heart and Lung Fitness
2. Muscle Toning Exercises

Activities such as walking, cycling, rowing or swimming performed over an extended period of time at a specific intensity all help improve the heart and lung (or cardiovascular/aerobic) fitness of our body. Add muscle toning exercises using your own body weight or hand weights with a healthy diet and you have the perfect combination for fat loss to occur.

Heart and Lung Fitness and Muscle Toning Exercises form a perfect partnership because together they help preserve muscle tissue and maximize fat loss potential. Maintaining muscle tissue is very important for women because it increases their metabolic rate and allows them to tone and reshape their body. Whereas, if weight is lost rapidly through dieting alone, the weight loss generally comes from muscle and fat. This may sound good, but I'm here as your personal coach to advise you different. The initial problem arises when you lose muscle because you are reducing your metabolic rate. Muscle loss, especially around the arms, chest and shoulder region also means that one is less likely to target the fat stores of the abdominal, butt and thigh regions. As a result, it becomes progressively harder to sustain any weight loss or a steady body weight and you get stuck with a pear-shaped body when looking in the mirror.

WW excels in transforming one's overall body shape by focusing on regaining body symmetry first. This revolutionary approach of strengthening the upper body muscles – arms, shoulders, back, chest and abdominals – is a unique aspect of the WW program that helps preserve muscle tissue in the upper body region whilst increasing one's resting metabolic rate (higher energy expenditure at rest) as the muscles tone and rebuild themselves. Combined with a regular heart and lung fitness exercise such as power walking and a healthy eating plan you have a unique approach that promotes fat burning activity of this normally dormant area.

Charting Your Progress

Establishing benchmarks and charting your progress is a great way to maintain motivation towards achieving your goal. Using various charts and logs helps identify improvements in

INTRODUCTION

health, fitness, body shape and well-being. Personal results are not just found on the scales. We know this because you can lose weight and still have a pear shaped body with protruding thighs.

By charting your progress you are compiling various aspects of performance about yourself that help maintain motivation. The ability to record and monitor your physical activity as well as Body Mass Index (BMI), body weight and body measurements, together with various medical tests involving blood glucose and cholesterol all help towards maintaining motivation and achieving your best body shape ever! Charting your progress will be outlined in more detail in Step 3.

Waistline Workout Success Story

To show you how WW works, let's follow the success of Karen, 38, a mother of two. Like a number of women, Karen was frustrated with dieting failures. Over the years she had put on weight, despite regular exercise and watching her fat intake. She has also been caught on the high protein, low carbohydrate fad that always led to her weight rebounding back on, plus some more, because all it was doing was creating nutrient deficiency. "The Waistline Workout Paul provided me with is something unique," says Karen. "It showed me the importance of consuming all the right nutrients as part of the recommended dietary intake for good health. It also provided me with an exercise plan with a specific focus for reducing my waistline and thighs. As a result, I knew what I was doing and when. With all the systems in place and a goal in mind I regained my body symmetry and look and feel great." Karen lost 14 kg (30 lbs) in 15 weeks and has gained a new body. More importantly, she learned the process that allowed her to strip inches from her hip, butt, thighs, waist, back and arms for a total body transformation. Let's see how below:

	Week 1	Week 5	Week 10	Week 15
Weight	79kg	75kg	69kg	65kg
BMI	29	27.5	25.5	23.8
Waistline	92cm	88cm	83.5cm	79cm
Hip/Thighs	106cm	101cm	95cm	89cm

In the initial weeks, weight loss may not seem very prominent. This is to be expected because muscle is developing whilst stripping body fat. As you will soon learn, muscle weighs more than fat and that is the reason why losing weight is not the short term focus. Instead you should be focusing on improvements in your lifestyle, diet and exercise routine and body composition. Through consistency and using a number of body measurements and visual aids such as photographs, motivation is kept high. Once, you reach the crucial 8-10 week mark, this is where real changes start too happen around the body. This is because you have allowed time for your body's internal chemistry (cell structure) to alter through proper nutrition, regular exercise and positive lifestyle changes. Ultimately, the Body Mass Index has reduced to the healthy BMI range between the score of 20-25 (see pages 55-56).

Visual Body Transformation

Through the visual power of photographs you can compare the body transformation from week 1 and 15. Notice the difference between the upper, mid and lower body regions and where the fat has been stripped away. The end result is what is referred to as obtaining good body symmetry – weighing less, better posture and poise, trimmer waist, sexier butt and thighs and much healthier body.

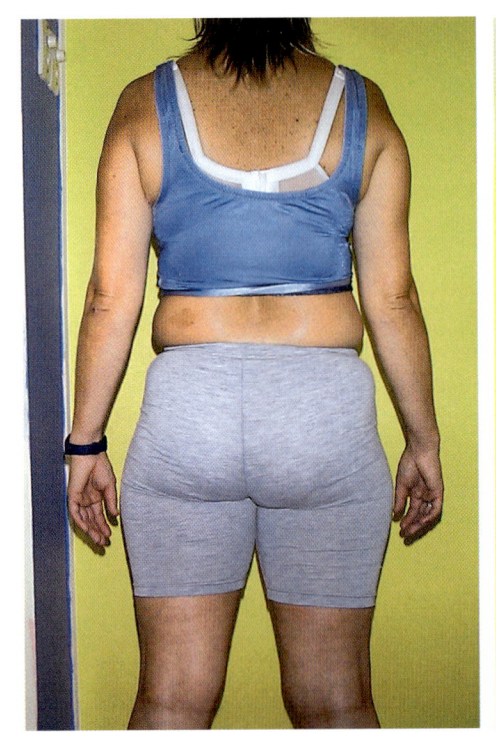

Starting out – Week 1

- Out of shape and overweight

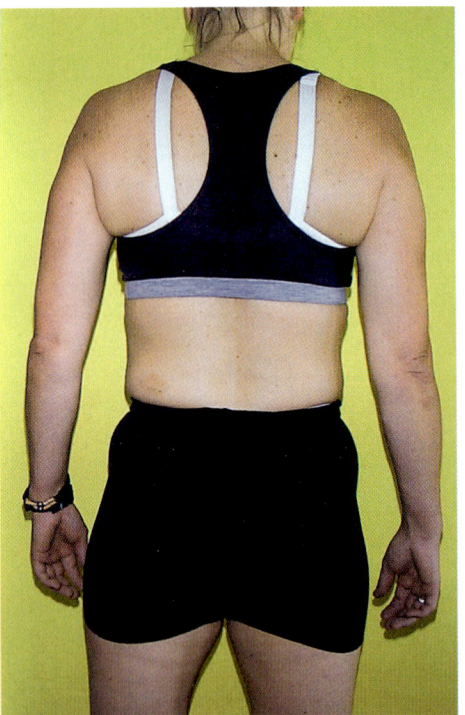

By Week 15

- Better body symmetry
- Lighter on the scales
- Improved posture
- Trimmer waistline
- Firmer and slimmer thighs
- More motivated

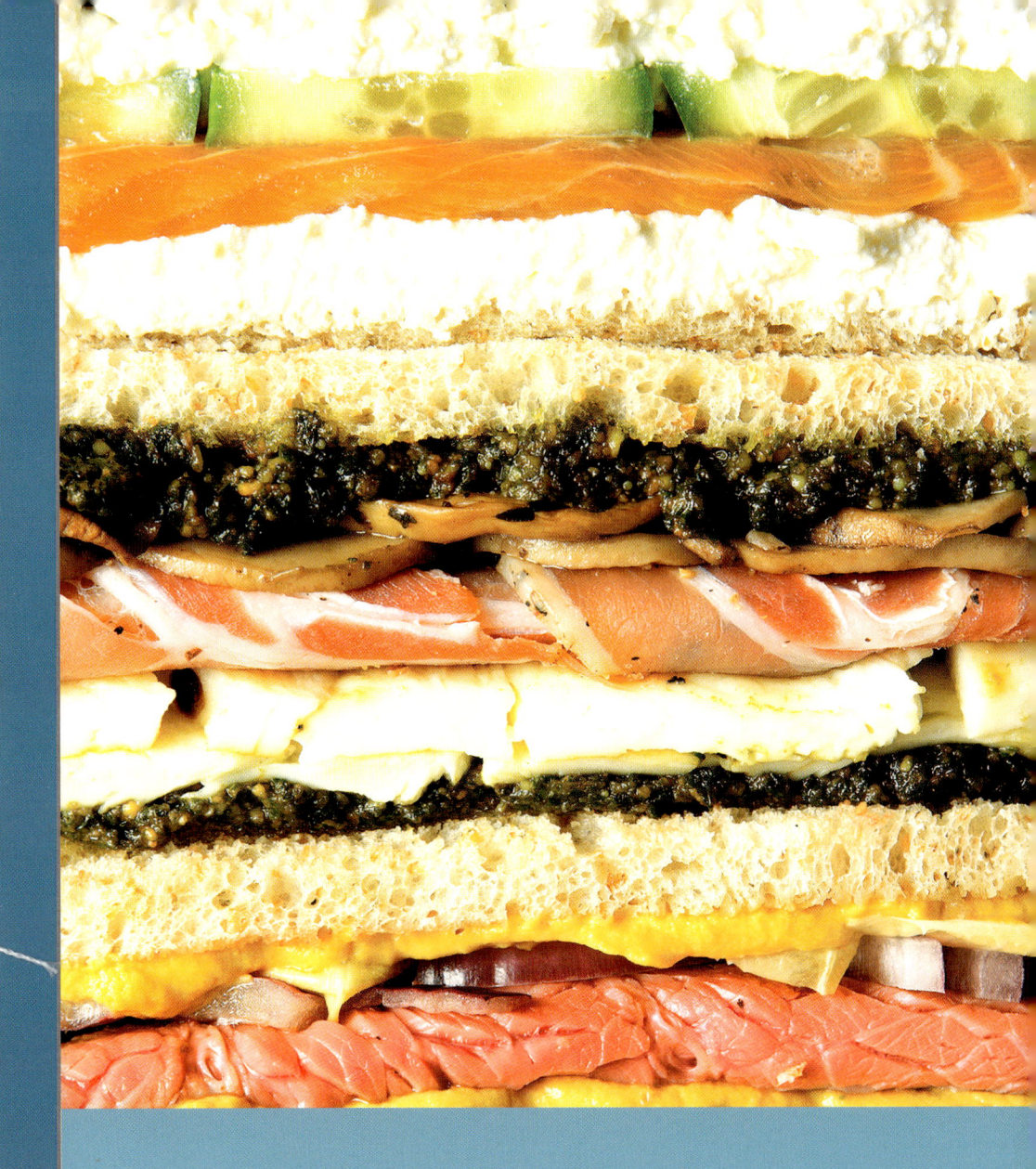

Step 1
Establishing a Healthy Eating Diet Plan
The RDI Diet Plan Approach

In this step you'll set out to establish a healthy eating diet plan using a Recommended Dietary Intake (RDI) Plan for good health.

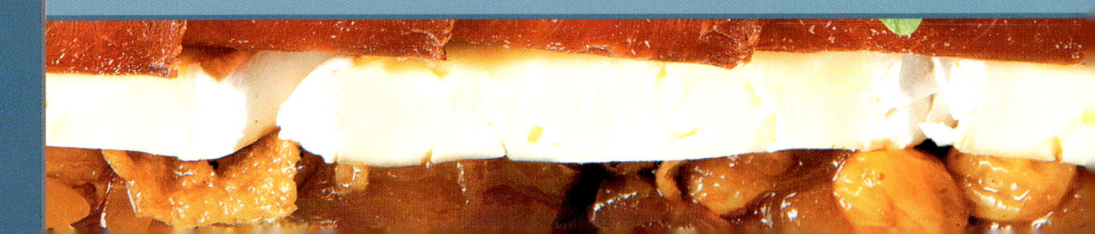

Importance of Losing Excess Weight

There are not many people who jump on the scales that are ever happy with their weight. Most people when asked believe they need to shed a few kilos and they are probably right because more than half the population is now regarded as overweight or obese. Being overweight has a number of health implications including increased risk of many diseases, particularly hypertension, cardiovascular disease and type 2 diabetes. Holding extra unwanted kilos on the body can place a tremendous strain on your heart and other bodily functions. It can also increase your blood pressure, compounding the risk of heart attack or stroke. So, as most people predict, losing a few kilos (pounds) can help prevent or help control these problems, especially if the extra fat being carried is around one's hips or waistline.

Moving away from the scales and looking into the mirror, many people may not like what they see. It has been observed that the area where you store fat first is also the area where you generally lose fat last. The body you are observing is often a result of poor dietary habits and chopping and changing between diet plans. Yet with the introduction of WW we aim to turn this around for you.

The WW Approach

Dieting alone can in fact make you fat by causing what is known as the yo-yo syndrome – a diet merry-go-round of losing weight, regaining it to lose it again, slowing one's metabolism. This is often because when losing weight through dieting alone, crucial muscular tissue is lost, primarily of the upper body region. Then, as the diet itself dissolves, this precious muscle fiber is hard to replace and often replaced with expanded fat cells. Many people tend to repeat this cycle over and over again. A resulting trimmer upper body and loss on the scales is now dubbed by a pear-shaped lower body that showcases the protruding thighs.

Various prime time magazines offering rapid weight loss success may be true in some instances, but you can be assured that you are only losing weight from the upper body region – face, chest, shoulders and arms – by way of losing lean muscle tissue and fluid loss that ultimately leads to larger looking thighs and a rebound effect as the plan can not be maintained.

WW has been developed as a result of these fundamentals. The objective is focusing on weight loss through combining the RDI of foods for good health along with specific exercises that aim to develop a more symmetrical body proportion - balancing the upper and lower body region - to ultimately make you look slimmer and trimmer all over. WW is therefore not a fad or short term fix; it is a long term plan for achieving better health and a trimmer body.

Ultimately, WW has been developed as a corrective weight loss plan for people who have reached a diet plateau with nowhere to go or disillusioned by the whole diet world. Even more importantly, WW is the corrective approach for women who have made mistakes and tried everything including starving themselves and now understand that what they have done up until now hasn't worked and whilst they may have lost weight and often regained it back again, the diets they have followed never seems to reduce the target areas long term.

Setting WW Apart from Others

With a million and one weight loss programs around, deciding which one is right for you is actually simpler than you think. I say this because if you turn your focus towards 'better health' as opposed to 'losing weight' you will begin to see how gaining the appropriate nutrients as part of the RDIs promoted by governments throughout the world are essential for good health. You begin to realize that diets you have followed in the past, such as high protein, low carbohydrate or low fat generally restrict important nutrients or create imbalances that may help lose weight quickly but eventually lead to lethargy, fatigue, cravings and even sickness and ultimately poor health and a rebound in weight and body fat. By restricting various nutrients or healthy food groups, people who are trying to lose weight can be at increased risk of deficiencies of a few key nutrients that help it run efficiently. Overtime, it gets harder and harder to lose weight which can have an affect on one's long-term health.

On the other hand, by eating foods from the recommended food groups that attract all the appropriate RDIs and choosing water as the choice of liquids over other commercial drinks, including alcohol and caffeine related drinks, the balance can then come from consuming the right portion sizes to meet your body's energy needs – it makes sense! My first weight loss book titled 'How to Lose Your Love Handles' provides this exact approach. The 3 Hour Rule® I developed for this book is a system of eating that shows you how to manage your RDIs over 5 smaller meals each day, approximately every 3 hours. This is great for people who need to maintain their blood sugar and energy levels and like a system or routine that ultimately leads to reducing their love handles.

As one size doesn't fit all, what WW now offers is a more flexible system of dieting that promotes the same ideals but is specific in targeting the hip, butt and waistline region. More specifically: WW shows you how to regain overall body symmetry.

Recommended Dietary Intakes (RDI)

To improve the health and well-being and reduce the risk of diet-related human disease, dietary guidelines have been established by various countries around the world that seek to promote the potential benefits of healthy eating. Designed on the basis of available scientific knowledge that is reviewed from time to time, Recommended Dietary Intakes (RDI) are the levels of intake of essential nutrients considered, in the judgement of expert committees within each government to be adequate to meet the known nutritional needs of practically all healthy people. Evidence is examined from human clinical studies and national eating patterns to arrive at recommended intakes for a variety of categories such as age and gender. You will find RDIs are now used as the basis in nutritional labelling on foods.

Daily intakes of essential nutrients (vitamins, minerals and protein) derived from estimates of requirements for each age and gender incorporate generous factors to accommodate variations in absorption and metabolism. Because there are many complex relationships between foods and nutrients, they can mutually influence the absorption, metabolism and retention of other nutrients. When a diet is well balanced and nutrients are in adequate supply, such interactions pose few problems. Although, when the intake of some nutrients is habitually low, excesses of others can have negative effects on the body. Most importantly, when a diet is designed to contain the relevant nutrients, it is more likely to contain all other dietary factors necessary for health that are not listed.

The following table (Table 1) of recommendations of nutrients adapted from the National Health and Medical Research Council (NHMRC) are intended as a guide for compiling diets from basic foods for women aged 18-54, 54+ as well as those pregnant and lactating. The RDIs here apply to those of average weight, height, activity and health and include a margin of safety to cover individual differences. As RDIs are based upon estimates of requirements that include a generous safety factor, you should always consult your doctor or nutritionist before starting to see if these meets your health needs, especially if pregnant or lactating. This table is then followed by a vitamin and mineral chart that helps you understand the exact types of foods with the RDI category itself.

Table 1: Recommended Dietary Intakes (RDI) for Women

	\[Women\] 19-54 yrs	54+ yrs	Pregnant	Lactating
Vitamin A	750	750	750	1200
Thiamin (mg)	0.8	0.7	1.0	1.2
Riboflavin (mg)	1.2	1.0	1.5	1.7
Niacin (mg)	13	11	15	18
Vitamin B-6 (mg)	0.9-1.4	0.8-1.1	0.9-1.6	1.6-2.2
Total Folate (µg)	200	200	400	350
Vitamin B-12 (µg)	2.0	2.0	3.0	2.5
Vitamin C (mg)	30	30	60	75
Vitamin E (mg)	7.0	7.0	7.0	9.5
Zinc (mg)	12	12	16	18
Iron (mg)	12-16	5-7	22-36	12-16
Iodine (µg)	120	120	150	170
Magnesium (mg)	270	270	300	340
Calcium (mg)	800	1000	1100	1200
Phosphorus (mg)	1000	1000	1200	1200
Selenium (µg)	70	70	80	85
Sodium (mmol)	40-100	40-100	40-100	40-100
(mg)	920-2300	920-2300	920-2300	920-2300
Potassium (mmol)	50-140	50-140	50-140	50-240
(mg)	1950-5460	1950-5460	+0	+0
Protein (g)	45	45	+6	+16
WATER	2 liters or more (8 x 250ml glasses per day)			

Source adapted from the National Health and Medical Research Council (NHMRC). Note: This table may be revised from time to time by the government to reflect the latest available scientific research findings.

Guidelines

- Recommendations for dietary intakes of vitamin D were not considered to be necessary unless people are housebound, since the vitamin D status is often determined by exposure to UV light from the sun. Warning: Too much sun increases the risk of skin cancer.
- Iron is expressed as a range to allow for differences in bioavailability of iron from different foods. The RDIs for pregnancy are for the 2nd and 3rd trimesters.
- Pregnancy and lactation increases the need for most nutrients as shown. The WW program itself is not designed for women who are pregnant or lactating, more so as an educational guide. Always follow your doctor's and nutritionist's advice.
- Many individuals may consume much less than the RDI for a nutrient without ill-effect because their individual requirement is also less.
- At present there is no evidence that excessive intakes of nutrients are beneficial, to the contrary they may well become toxic – this is another reason why RDIs are carefully set to fall well below the toxic threshold for any known nutrient.
- The RDI for energy is different as it must relate more specifically to the need of the individual in order to avoid being underweight or obese.

RDI Vitamin and Mineral Chart

Your body needs vitamins to help it metabolize amino acids, carbohydrates and fats. Your body also needs an adequate supply of minerals for a multitude of functions. When minerals are obtained directly from natural plant sources – *fruit, vegetables, legumes, whole grains, nuts and seeds* – the mineral elements are compatible with the human body, ensuring effective digestion, absorption and utilization for rebuilding, regulation and protection. The following table (Table 2) outlines the essential vitamins and minerals for good health.

Table 2: Good sources of the most essential vitamins and minerals are:

Vitamin/Mineral	Food Sources	Role
Vitamin A Retinol	Liver, fortified milk.	Essential for eyes, skin and the proper function of the immune system. Helps maintain hair, bones and teeth.
Vitamin A - Beta Carotene	Carrots, squash, broccoli, green leafy vegetables.	Antioxidant. Converted to Vitamin A in the body.
Vitamin B1 (Thiamine)	Sunflower seeds, pork, whole and enriched grains, dried beans.	Necessary for carbohydrate metabolism and muscle coordination. Promotes proper nerve function.

Vitamin B2 (Riboflavin)	Liver, milk, spinach, enriched noodles, mushrooms.	Needed for metabolism of all foods and the release of energy to cells. Essential to the functioning of Vitamin B6 and Niacin.
Vitamin B3 (Niacin)	Mushrooms, bran, tuna, chicken, beef, peanuts, enriched grains.	Needed in many enzymes that convert food to energy. Helps maintain a healthy digestive tract and nervous system. In very large doses, lowers cholesterol (large doses should only be taken under the advice of a physician).
Vitamin B6	Animal protein foods, spinach, broccoli, bananas.	Needed for protein metabolism and absorption, carbohydrate metabolism. Helps form red blood cells. Promotes nerve and brain function.
Folic Acid (Folate)	Green, leafy vegetables, orange juice, organ meats, sprouts.	Essential for the manufacture of genetic material as well as protein metabolism and red blood cell formation.
Vitamin B12	Found almost exclusively in animal products.	Builds genetic material. Helps form red blood cells.
Vitamin C	Citrus fruits, paw paw, kiwi fruit, broccoli, potatoes, capsicum, brussels sprouts, cauliflower, cabbage strawberries, broccoli, green peppers.	Antioxidant. Helps bind cells together and strengthens blood vessel walls. Helps maintain healthy gums. Aids in the absorption of iron.
Vitamin E	Corn or cottonseed oil, butter, brown rice, soybean oil, vegetable oils such as corn, cottonseed or soybean, nuts, wheat germ.	Antioxidant. Helps form red blood cells, muscles and other tissues. Preserves fatty acids.
Zinc	Oysters, shrimp, crab, beef, turkey, whole grains, peanuts, beans.	Necessary element in more than 100 enzymes that are essential to digestion and metabolism.
Iron	Liver, lean meats, kidney beans, enriched bread, raisins. **Note:** Oxalic acid in spinach hinders iron absorption.	Essential for making haemoglobin, the red substance in blood that carries oxygen to body cells.

Iodine	Asparagus, blueberry, cucumber, peanut, spinach, strawberry, turnip, watermelon.	Essential for regulating the thyroid gland in its purpose to control the body's metabolism.
Magnesium	Spinach, beet greens, broccoli, tofu, popcorn, cashews, wheat bran.	Activates enzymes needed to release energy in body. Needed by cells for genetic material and bone growth.
Calcium	Dairy milk, yogurt, cheese; broccoli, sardines, turnip greens. If you are lactose intolerant or allergic to dairy, good calcium sources are nuts (especially almonds), salmon, calcium fortified low fat soy milk.	Helps build strong bones and teeth. Promotes muscle and nerve function. Helps activate enzymes needed to convert food to energy.
Phosphorus	Chicken breast, milk, lentils, egg yolks, nuts, cheese.	With calcium builds bones and teeth. Needed for metabolism, body chemistry, nerve and muscle function.
Selenium	Adequate amounts are found in seafood, kidney, liver and other meats. Grains and other seeds contain varying amounts depending on the soil content.	Antioxidant. Interacts with Vitamin E to prevent breakdown of fats and body chemicals.
Sodium	Artichoke, beetroot, cabbage, carrot, cashew, celery, chick pea, coconut, garlic, kale, kelp, lentil, olives, parsley, radish, sunflower seed, turnip, watercress, white beans.	Essential for production of saliva, maintenance of normal blood pressure and maintaining the correct water balance between cells. Note: Common household table salt is inorganic (chloride) which can be harmful to the kidneys, raise blood pressure and promote hardening of the arteries. Sodium is only valuable when it's organic and balanced.
Potassium	Peanuts, bananas, orange juice, green beans, mushrooms, oranges, broccoli, sunflower seeds.	Helps maintain regular fluid balance. Needed for nerve and muscle function.

Protein		
A – Animal	A – meat, poultry, fish, eggs	Amino acids are the foundation of all protein. Amino acids are the building blocks of human cells and living tissues. All the essential amino acids required for the maintenance of life are obtainable from: meat, poultry, fish, dairy, eggs, nuts, seeds, legumes, whole grains. (Protein sources are also related to Zinc, Iron and Calcium)
P – Plant	P – nuts, seeds, peas, beans, legumes, soya	
C – Calcium	C – milk, yogurt, cheese.	

Note: Although not all vitamins and minerals are referred to as part of the RDI chart, the majority of these can be found in those food sources mentioned above.

Energy Balance – Variety versus Over-consumption

As variety in a diet increases, it is important to control serving sizes, the amounts of each food eaten and the overall portion sizes to avoid over-consumption of energy and thus avoid obesity. Portion sizes are important because larger portions usually contain more calories (kilojoules). If you eat more calories than your body needs, you will put on weight. Whereas, if you eat less calories and work within the recommended dietary intake range, you'll lose weight, especially when moderate-intensity exercise is performed regularly and you start drinking more water. More importantly, you'll be looking after your long term health.

Taking control of your serving sizes and overall food intake (portion size) is essential for controlling your weight. A portion is the total amount of food you choose to eat at one sitting. Reducing the overall portion sizes of your meals will reduce the total energy intake, so going back for seconds should become a thing of the past. The other ideal to consider in this equation is that foods often of the same weight and size can be totally different in calories. Take a 200 gram apple and 200 gram piece of chocolate – the calorie difference is in the thousands. So understanding energy balance plays a vital role in your daily food choices.

RDI – Food Translation

The Recommended Dietary Intake (RDI) is the backbone of the Food Pyramid and recommended serving sizes. For an easy comprehension and familiarity with these foods groups, WW goes one step further to translate this into a chart outlining the 3 major food groups – Carbohydrates, Protein and Fat (plus water which is essential fluid for life) – and the relevant portion sizes to satisfy the RDIs. Further subcategories are defined to ensure a wide variety of foods are chosen and all essential vitamins and minerals are met each day.

Food Group	Meal Portions
Complex Carbohydrates (Fiber)	
• Cereals and grains	• 4 portions a day Active people may need more.
• Vegetables and salads	• 4 portions a day Active people may need more.
• Fruits	• 1–2 portions a day
Protein	
• Protein (A) animal source	• 1–2 lean portions a day (depending on body weight and energy requirements)
• Protein (P) plant source	• 1 portion a day
• Protein (C) calcium source	• 2 portions a day
Fats (Lipids)	
• Oils and margarines • Generally no extra dietary fats are needed if consuming the Recommended Daily Intake of Protein (A,P,C) portions provided. • Always be aware of the hidden fats in pre-cooked meals, packaged foods and restaurant meals.	• One tablespoon per day For example: If you consume the following foods you will not need any extra fat in your diet. • Protein (A) – at least three portions of fish per week; 4 servings of lean meats • Protein (P) – mixed nuts/seeds • 60g avocado
Water (H20)	Drink 2 liters (or 8 glasses) of water a day. More if you exercise.

Source: Adapted from the Dietary Guidelines for Australians (NHMRC)

Now that you've learnt this background information, designing your meals will become much simpler to control because there's now some sense to what you are doing. The range in serving sizes often used (i.e. 1-3 servings) simply refers to one's energy demands. The lower one's energy demands, the lower the serving size and visa versa. By applying the Body Coach® Daily Food Portion Chart on page 36-37, you will achieve the right balance of these 3 major food groups described in more detail below.

Familiar Nutrition Terms

In more familiar terms, the essential vitamins and minerals that form part of the Recommended Dietary Intake and Food Pyramid consist primarily of three (3) major food groups commonly referred to as:

1. Carbohydrate
2. Protein
3. Fat

Carbohydrate

Carbohydrates consist of starch, sugars and some components of fiber. Sugars are the simplest form of carbohydrate; starches are complex carbohydrates which are broken down to sugars during digestion. Carbohydrates are the most important fuel of the body and should make up to 50 percent of one's energy intake. Starch and sugars supply 4 calories (16 kilojoules) per gram, fiber supplies less depending on how much is digested. Carbohydrates are found in plant foods such as cereals – wholegrain bread, brown rice and high-fiber cereals including oats; vegetables, legumes (peas, beans, lentils) and fruit as well as low-fat dairy products in the form of lactose (milk and yoghurt). Balancing carbohydrates out throughout the day with protein and fat is important, as consuming carbohydrates alone or consuming too much can lead to various deficiencies and even bloating. This is often the case when an athlete stops training and continues to consume a similar amount of carbohydrates that the body doesn't require. Also be conscious here, as soft drinks, energy drinks and sports drinks add many unwanted sugars into the equation that can lead to bloating and even gas. So, unless you're an elite athlete playing intense sport for more than 30 minutes, stick to water and focus on cereals and grains, vegetables and salads and fruits as your preferred choice. Vegetables themselves should contribute a large proportion of the daily carbohydrate intake

Protein

Protein is vital for life because it supplies the body with essential amino acids required for growth, maintenance and renewal of body tissues including muscle, skin, bones, organs, nails and hair. Protein is a necessary constituent of all living cells and is continuously turned over. As the body can only store a small pool of amino acids, we must replace them regularly through a protein rich diet. As a percentage of the diet, protein should be around 20-30 percent of the total calories (kilojoules) consumed. Proteins supply 4 calories (16 kilojoules) per gram.

Protein requirements are generally calculated at 1 gram per kilogram of bodyweight. For example: a 70kg person requires 70 grams of usable protein. Athletes may require more. In food terms, usable protein refers to the amount of actual protein source found within a food. A 120 gram piece of beef, chicken or lamb for example has approximately 20 grams of useable protein. Other examples of useable proteins include:

- 1 egg = 4 grams
- 1 cup of oatmeal = 6 grams
- 25 grams of nuts = 10 grams
- 90 grams of tofu = 10 grams
- 1 cup of cottage cheese = 20 grams
- 100 grams of canned tuna = 25 grams
- 160 grams of fresh fish = 20 grams

A complete protein containing all the essential amino acids the body needs to consume include: eggs, cheese, milk, poultry, meat and fish – commonly found in animal and some plant sources. Other forms of proteins are derived from plant sources, which need to be combined with other sources to become a complete source and consumed within the same day. Plant sources include: grains, legumes, nuts and seeds. The combination for a complete protein source can be found when combining food sources such as: rice and soya beans; beans, rice and corn; hummus and tabouli; almonds, brasil and cashew nut combination; rice and lentils; porridge and soy milk, to name a few. For simplicity, I have broken Protein into three areas, which are described in more details in the following pages:

1. **Protein (A) – Animal Source**

2. **Protein (P) – Plant Source**

3. **Protein (C) – Calcium Source**

One should avoid protein in excess as it creates undesirable end products which can lead to kidney and liver problems, fluid imbalance and constipation and increased risk of Osteoporosis. On the other hand, protein deficiency can lead to tiredness and lethargy, lack of strength, bloating and poor digestion, irritability, tooth decay, frequent infections such as cold and flu, poor wound healing and the like. So be sure to keep a good protein balance through a good mixture of complete protein sources

Fat (Lipids)

Fats provide more than twice the energy per gram as either carbohydrate or protein, supplying 9 calories (or 37 Kilojoules) per gram. Most experts recommend that only 30 percent or less of the total calories be consumed as fat, with 20 percent from poly- and monounsaturated fats and 10 percent or less from saturated fats. Fats are oily or waxy substances made up of fatty acids and glycerol and cholesterol. If you eat a wide variety of naturally prepared foods such as fish, nuts and avocado, you will maintain your body's requirements of healthy fats. On the other hand, over-consumption of saturated fats found mainly in animal foods such as marbled beef, pork, butter, whole milk, egg yolks and hard cheese, can raise cholesterol levels.

Saturated fats also occur in some plant foods, such as cocoa butter, palm oil and coconut oil, and form the basis of many foods found on supermarket shelves and in takeaway foods outlets. The most hazardous fats are those unseen fats found mostly in commercially baked, fried or manufactured foods and easily added during preparation and cooking. Remember, most takeaway foods are fried, cooked or prepared in fat.

Commercially baked products, pastries, biscuits, cakes and sweets can also be high in saturated fat and sugar, since both act as a preservative. Be wary of accompaniments to your meals. Sauces made from cream, coconut, lard, mayonnaise, vegetable oils and butter are all high in fat. So, unless the overall fat intake is monitored, excess fats can contribute towards becoming overweight, heart disease and certain cancers. Whereas, consuming natural fats found in fish and nuts and seeds can assist in preventing some aspects of heart disease as long as the overall portion sizes are kept under control.

You can monitor the fat content of your foods by learning about foods that contain fat and how to reduce and replace them. This is why I place so much emphasis on foods containing complex carbohydrates (fiber) and a mixture of protein sources (A, P, C) that are low in fat.

Water

Water is the most essential of all nutrients, because without it one could not survive more than a few days. Around 2-3 liters of fluid are lost from the body each day and need to be replaced. Water is found in foods such as fruit, vegetables and salads, but most needs to be acquired from the clear natural source to the tune of 8 glasses or 2 liters a day. Most importantly, water is calorie free! Drinks such as herbal or green tea, coffee, red wine, diet soft drinks and cordials and even water based soups can contribute to your daily fluid intake. But caution should be taken for some of these drinks due to ingredients such as caffeine, sugar, alcohol and even sodium as they can add to your energy intake. To achieve the recommended 2 liters of water (8 glasses) a day, plus extra if exercising, the following information provides a helpful guideline to meet your needs:

- Water = 4 or more glasses
- Milk = 1-2 glasses
- Fruit / vegetable juice = 1 glass
- Green or herbal tea = 1-2 glasses
- Coffee = 1 glass (cup)
- Water based soup = 2 glasses
- Wine = 0-1 glass per day (not suitable for persons under 18)

Portion Sizes

Portion sizes are important in the diet equation because larger portions usually contain more calories (kilojoules). In simple terms, if you eat more calories than your body needs you will put on weight; if you eat less than your body needs you will lose weight. The following outline of essential nutrients and portion sizes will help manage your day better and keep you on track in your quest to reduce your body fat levels.

STEP 1

Complex Carbohydrate (Fiber) Food Sources Include:

Cereal and Grains – 4 portions a day (Active people may need more).
One portion equates to:

Wholegrain cereals and grains
- 1 cup (30–40 grams) wholegrain breakfast cereal (low sugar and salt)
- 1/3 cup of muesli (due to weight and density)
- 1 cup of oats (porridge)
- 1 cup of cooked basmati or jasmine rice (low in starch)
- 1 cup of cooked brown rice
- 1 cup of cooked wholemeal pasta
- 1 cup of barley, millet or buckwheat

Wholegrain breads
- 1 slice of wholegrain bread
- 1 slice of yeast-free bread
- 1/2 English muffin
- 1/2 pita bread
- 1 small wholegrain roll
- 1 corn tortilla

Legumes
- See Protein (P) plant

© fotolia, Blue-Fox

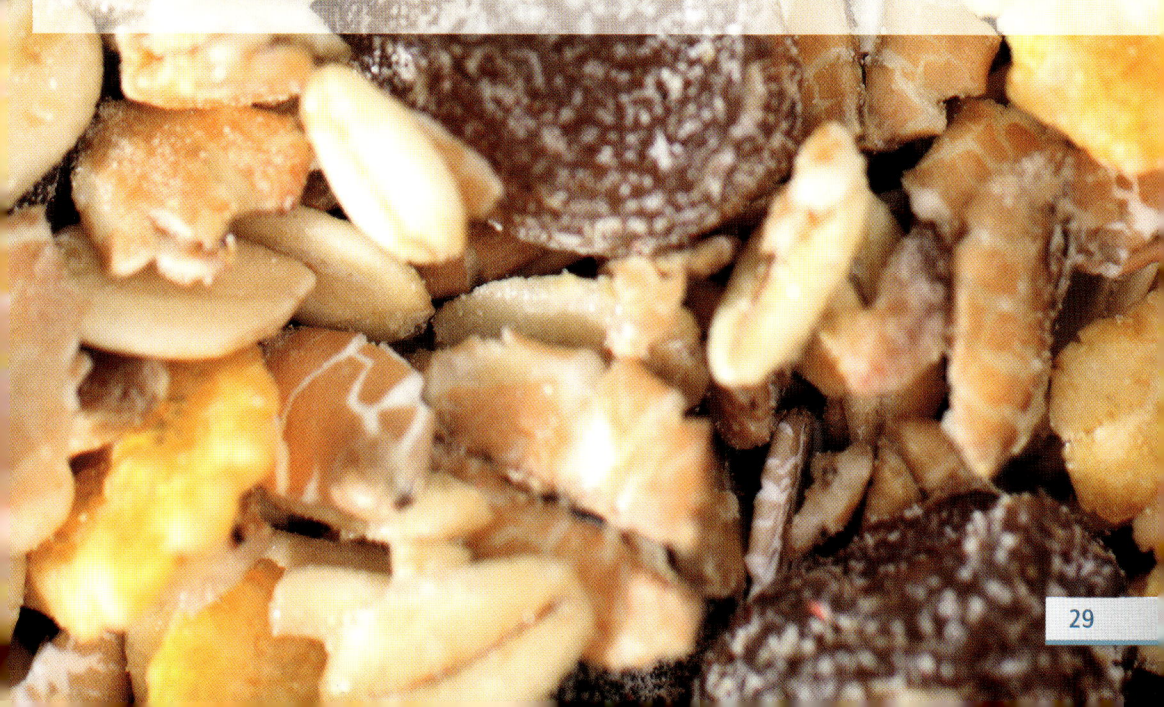

WAISTLINE WORKOUT

VEGETABLES and SALADS – 4 portions a day. Active people may need more. One portion (cooked) equals:

Flowering and green leafy vegetables
- 1/2 cup broccoli, asparagus, Brussels sprouts, cabbage, spinach, celery, bean sprouts, bok choy, watercress, all types of lettuce and cauliflower

Starchy vegetables
- 1 medium cooked potato or parsnip (1/2 cup)
- 1 piece pumpkin or sweet potato, the size of a medium potato (1/2 cup)

Colored vegetables
1/2 cup of (example not limited to):
- **Orange:** carrots, pumpkin
- **Yellow:** squash, capsicum
- **Green:** broccoli, spinach
- **Red:** capsicum, tomato (acid fruit)
- **White:** cauliflower, turnip

Salads
- 1 cup of mixed lettuce or salad vegetables including, but not limited to, alfalfa sprouts, beetroot, cabbage, capsicum, celery, cucumber, eggplant, radishes, tomato and snow peas

Other vegetables (including legumes)
- 1/2 cup of: broad beans, green beans, peas, zucchini, corn

© fotolia, Laure

STEP 1

FRUIT – 1-2 portions a day. A portion is generally understood to mean a piece of fruit the size of a tennis ball, diced loosely into a cup (about 150 grams). Note: fruit juice should be limited to 125 ml at a time because it is such a concentrated source of sugar.

Stone fruits
- Apples, apricots, blueberries, pears, cherries, grapes, paw paw, peaches, lychees, raspberries, strawberries

Sweet fruits
- Bananas, dates, figs, prunes, raisins, dried fruits

Acid fruits
- Grapefruits, limes, kiwi fruits, oranges, lemons, pineapples, mandarins, tomatoes, passionfruit

© fotolia, Elenathewise

Proteins

For a good selection of proteins in your diet, I have broken them down into three key areas:
1. Animal source (A)
2. Plant source (P)
3. Calcium source (C)

Protein (A) animal source
1–2 lean portions a day (100–200 grams). Active people may need more.

Meat (at least 4 portions a week)
- 100 grams of cooked lean red meat (e.g. beef, lamb)
- 80 grams of shaved and unprocessed lean red meat
- 2 slices of roast

Poultry
- 100 grams of cooked skinless chicken breast
- 100 grams of lean chicken strips
- 100 grams of lean turkey breast or lean turkey chops
- 100 grams of shaved and unprocessed chicken or turkey breast

Fish and shellfish (at least 3 portions a week)
- 120 grams of white fish filet
- 100 grams of salmon filet
- 100 grams of canned fish: tuna, salmon, sardines
- 100 grams of crab, lobster, scallops or prawns

Eggs
- 1 large whole egg
- 2 egg whites

STEP 1

Protein (P) Plant Source
- 1 portion per day, or at least every second day

Nuts and seeds
- Mixed nuts and seeds: raw or blanched almonds, brazil nuts and cashews; sesame, sunflower or pepita seeds. (1 portion of raw nuts or seeds = 30 grams, or about the size of a golf ball)
- 1 teaspoon of peanut or almond spread

Beans and peas (legumes)
- 1/3 cup of cooked kidney beans, split peas, chick peas or other dried beans
- 1/3 cup of cooked lentils
- 1/2 cup (220g) cooked canned (baked) beans
- 1/4 cup of low-fat hummus

Soya
- 1/3 cup cooked soya beans
- 100 grams of tofu

Plant proteins are incomplete proteins and need to be combined to complement each other, for example, rice with beans or a mixture of various nuts. This is especially important for vegetarians.

© fotolia, Svetlana Lukienko

WAISTLINE WORKOUT

Protein (C) Calcium Source
- 2 portions a day

Milk
- 1 cup (250ml) of reduced-fat milk (fresh, long-life or reconstituted)
- 1 cup (250ml) of calcium-fortified low-fat soy milk

Yoghurt
- 200 gram tub of low-fat yoghurt
- 200 gram tub of natural fruit yoghurt with friendly bacteria
- 150ml yoghurt drink

Cheese
- 20–40 grams of low-fat cheese
- 1–2 slices of low-fat cheese
- 1/4 cup of shredded low-fat tasty cheese
- 50–100 grams of low-fat cottage or ricotta cheese

Note: If you are lactose intolerant or allergic to dairy, good calcium sources are:
- Nuts, especially almonds
- Fresh or tinned salmon, bones and all
- Calcium-fortified low-fat soy milk

© fotolia, Tomo Jesenicnik

Fat (Lipids)

If consuming the recommended daily intake of Protein (APC) portions provided above, generally no extra dietary fats are needed. For instance, if consuming:

- Protein (A) – at least three portions of fish per week or four servings of lean meats and eggs
- Protein (P) – 30 grams of mixed nuts and/or seeds each day
- 60g avocado
- 1 tablespoon of oil or margarine

What's more important in the case of fat is being aware of the hidden fats in pre-cooked meals and packaged foods including chocolate, cookies, chips and other treats. Also be aware of the way meals are prepared in relation to the oils and sauces, cooking or frying methods in restaurants, fast food outlets and at home.

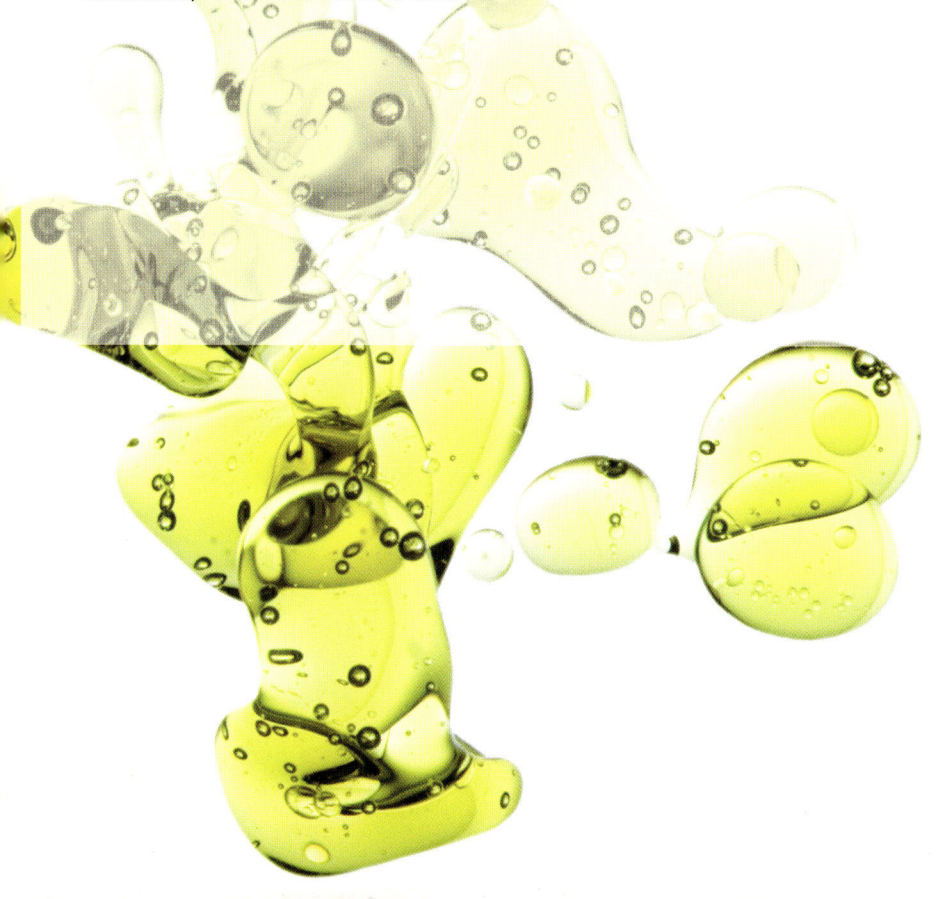

Body Coach® Daily Food Portion Chart

My goal from the onset has been to educate you by showing you the links between the various Recommended Dietary Intakes (RDI) and food groups – Carbohydrates, Proteins, Fat – and Water. For easy management, the above information has now been transferred into a simplified eating model referred to as the Body Coach® Daily Food Portion Chart which we will work from. This chart is broken into two parts:

(1) Food portions - on the left side
(2) Extra foods for active people - on the right

Fulfilling the 'food portion' requirements on the left is your number one priority for gaining all the RDIs. Throughout the wider community this is often referred to as 'eating a wide variety of foods in moderation'. But without proper guidance this phrase can easily be misunderstood. So, keeping to the left of the chart is your priority. Any extra foods consumed due to energy requirements should come from those food groups boxed on the right side of the chart. In order to ensure consistency and enable you to monitor, assess and improve your eating patterns, any additional foods that are consumed but do not fall within the food category portions promoted should be recorded at the bottom of the chart.

WW understands there are many social aspects of life to enjoy. Therefore, consistency with this plan is promoted over perfection. The main objective is to improve where you stand today in terms of the variety of foods consumed on a daily basis. The helps you control your portion sizes and your food energy intake. It also helps you change bad habits and make good ones stick. Making the right food choices is important for maintaining a healthy weight range and long-term well-being.

The numbered boxes under the heading 'Food Portions' are the portions of each food group you need to base your meals around. Cross off or shade in the boxes as you plan your meals or as you consume food throughout the day. The numbered boxes under the heading 'Extras' on the right side of the chart are for extra food energy choices for active people. Choose your extra foods from the food groups supplied on the chart.

The Body Coach® Daily Food Portion Chart can be used to help you plan meals ahead of time or make health meal choices throughout the day, even if you purchase your meals. Apply the following chart to manage your daily food intake and routine (copy chart page as necessary):

STEP 1

Body Coach® Daily Food Portion Chart

Complex Carbohydrates (fiber)	Food Portions				Extra foods – for active people			
Cereals & Grains	1	2	3	4	5	6	7	8
Vegetables & Salads	1	2	3	4	5	6	7	8
Fruit			1	2	3			

Protein								
Animal (A)			1	2	3			
Plant (P)				1	2			
Calcium (C)			1	2	3			

Fat								
1 tablespoon of oil or margarine				1				
For every protein (A or P) source shade in one box	1	2	3					

Water (250ml Glasses)	1	2	3	4				
	5	6	7	8	9	10	11	12

Record any additional foods (or drinks) consumed below:

_____

_____

Note: Use this information to gauge your habits and making healthier food choices. Always work with your doctor to ensure the right eating plan for you. If you find yourself consuming excess of only one or two types of food, you are limiting essential nutrients and you will need to shift your eating patterns to a more balanced approach that focuses on achieving all the RDIs.

WAISTLINE WORKOUT

Sample RDI Eating Day

By breaking the day into 3 meals and 2 snacks (or 5 smaller meals a day approximately every 3 hours), you are providing a consistent supply of food and energy in controlled portions that digest easier and help maintain balanced blood sugar levels throughout the day – significant for those with diabetes. This is important to understand, because long gaps between meals or large meals which can lead to long gaps can result in energy slumps and cravings, a feature many people may have experienced in the afternoons. Consuming smaller meals more often also allows you to gain all the appropriate RDIs and is the basis of the example below. Although, 3–6 meals a day is okay. The objective is to control the portion size and feel satisfied without over consuming unwanted calories and energy and focus on drinking more water as the choice liquid and consuming more vegetables.

Sample RDI Eating – including 8 glasses of water

Breakfast
- 1 cup of bran cereal and low-fat milk; 1 piece of wholegrain toast spread with peanut butter; 1 glass of water; 1 cup of green tea.

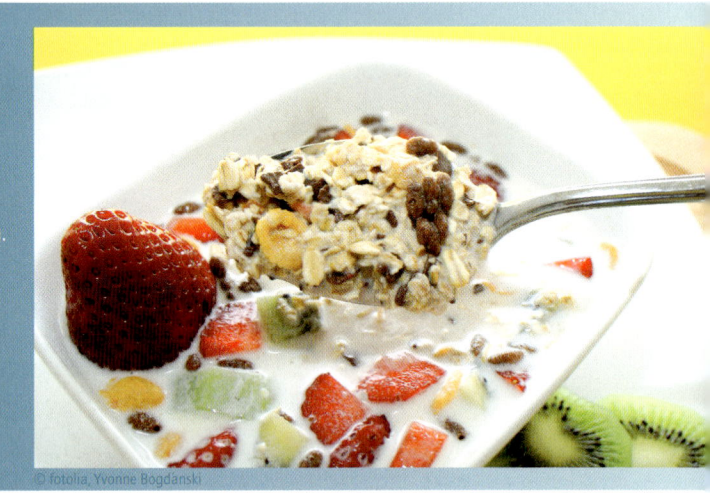

Snack
- 1 tub of low-fat yoghurt; 1 piece of fruit; 1 glass of water

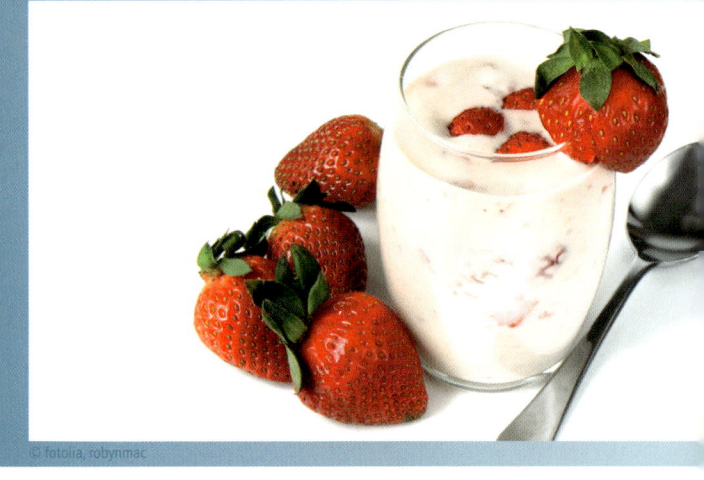

STEP 1

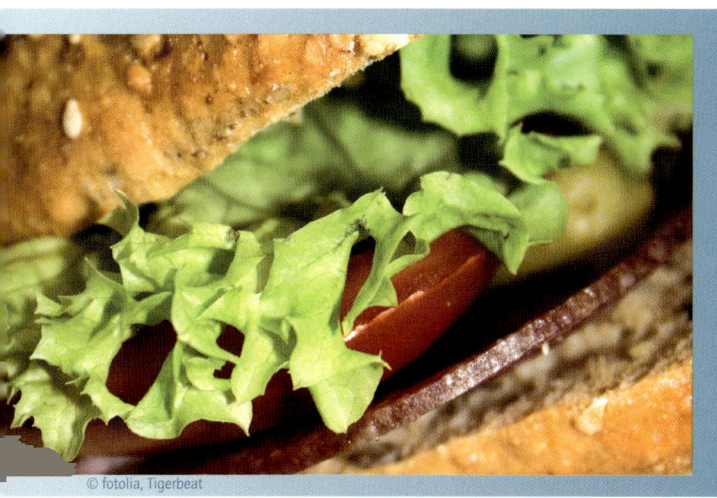

Lunch
- Lean meat and salad sandwich (2 slices of wholegrain bread; 30g of avocado as spread; 100g of lean meat; 1 cup of mixed salad); 1-2 glasses of water

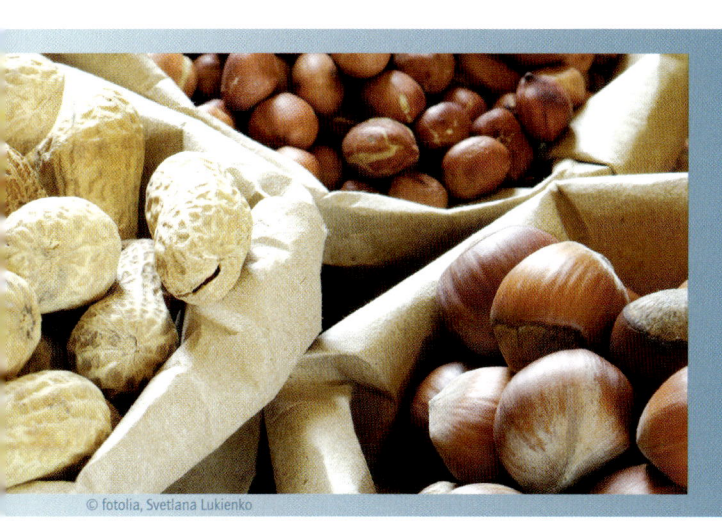

Afternoon Snack
- 20-30 grams of mixed raw nuts; 1 glass of water

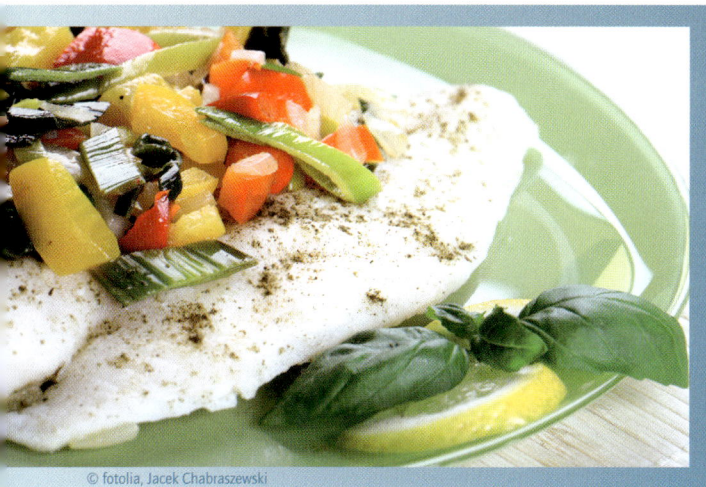

Dinner
- 160 grams of steamed fish, 1 cup of brown rice and cooked mixed vegetables with teaspoon of olive oil; 1 bowl of mixed salad; 200g of low-fat custard with 1 diced banana for dessert; 1-2 glasses of water

Similar Energy, Different Sizes

Here I've compiled information about foods with similar energy levels (i.e. calories) but different sizes. In many instances, you will find similar sizes being referred to in relation to portion sizes, for instance – 250 ml or 1 cup is a prime example. But a cup of salad is not the same as a cup of vegetables – they are different in weight and in energy density. If we were to compare a 100 gram chocolate bar with the amount of apples you could eat, it would equate to 8 medium size apples for the same energy level. With this example alone, you can see how easy it is to consume extra calories without knowing it and put on weight. A calorie counting book can help you further identify these. In the meantime, our goal is to focus on what you should be eating, rather than what you shouldn't be. The following examples are designed to help provide you with a good understanding between food groups containing the same energy value but different portion sizes.

PROTEINS

A and P – Protein
- 100 grams of cooked lean meat
- 2 slices of roast meat
- 120 grams of fish
- 1/3 cup of mixed raw nuts
- 2 small eggs—scrambled, boiled, poached or in an omelette
- 100 grams of tinned fish—tuna, salmon, sardines
- 1 fish finger (25 grams)

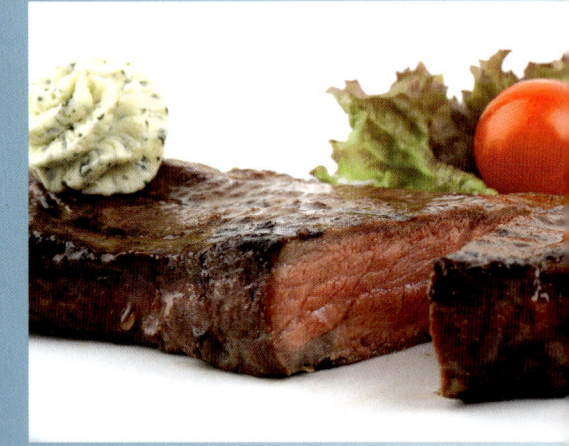

© fotolia, ChristianSchwier.de

C – Protein
- 200 gram carton of low-fat yoghurt (plain or fruit)
- 40 grams or 2 single slices of low-fat cheese
- 1 cup (250ml) of reduced fat cow's milk or goat's milk
- 1 cup (250ml) of lite soy milk fortified with calcium
- 1/2 cup (125ml) of low-fat custard
- 1/3 cup shredded low-fat tasty cheese
- 100 grams of salmon (and bones)

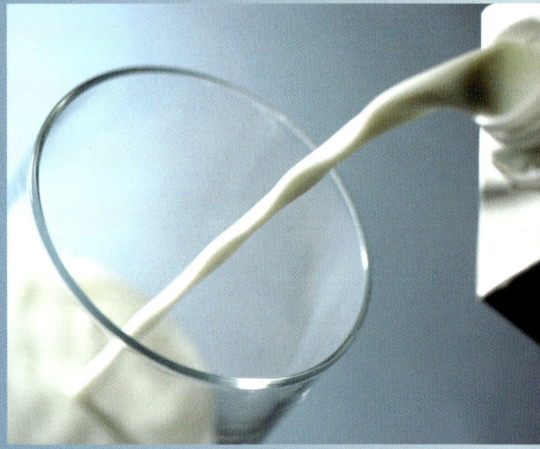

© fotolia, Anca Moanta

STEP 1

COMPLEX CARBOHYDRATES (fiber)

Vegetables and salad
- 1 cup of mixed salad vegetables
- 1/2 cup of cooked vegetables
- 1 small potato

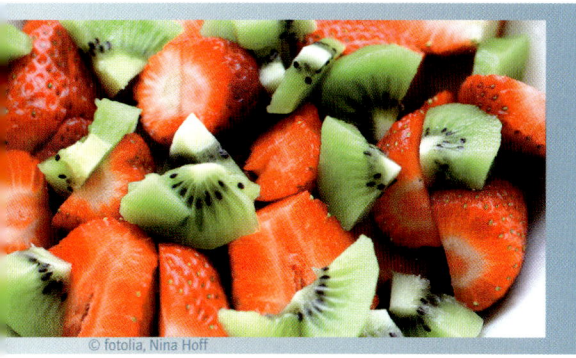

Fruit
- 1 medium (150 grams) piece of fruit—apple, pear
- 1 cup of freshly prepared mixed fruit salad
- 1/2 cup (125ml) of freshly squeezed fruit juice
- 2 small (total 150 grams) pieces of fruit—apricots, plums, figs
- 3–4 dried apricots

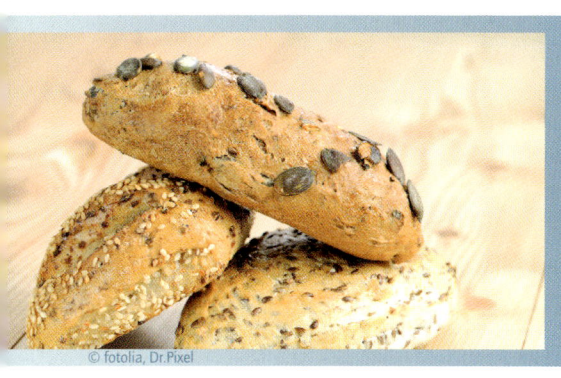

Bread, rice, pasta, noodles (preferably whole grain)
- 2 slices of wholegrain bread
- 1 medium wholegrain bread roll
- 1 small pita bread
- 3 crispbreads or 2 wheat biscuits
- 1 wholegrain muffin
- 1 cup (180 grams) of cooked rice, pasta/spaghetti, noodles

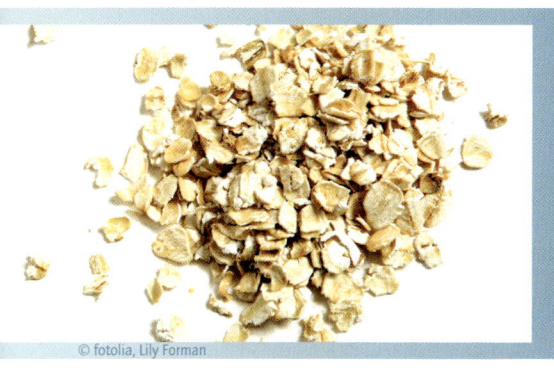

Cereals and grains (preferably whole grain)
- 1 cup (40 grams) of breakfast cereal (no added sugar)
- 1/2 cup (65 grams) of untoasted (natural) muesli
- 1 cup (230 grams) of cooked oats (porridge)

Talking about Alcohol

Firstly, there's nothing wrong with the occasional glass of red wine or beer as it plays an essential role in social interaction and psychological well-being. What you need to know though is that alcoholic drinks such as wine, beer and spirits contribute to your overall energy (calorie) including the mixers with the spirits such as soft drinks or fruit juices. This is because they supply alcoholic sugars that are high in energy but low in significant nutrients like vitamins and minerals. Drinking too much too often can lead to malnutrition, as the body is being starved of the essential nutrients found in natural foods. So, don't be fooled by people who are thin and consume alcohol regularly because they run a high risk of developing many cancers and malfunctions of the immune system.

It's no secret that some habits are hard to change, but this one is important because we need to focus on gaining all the recommended dietary intakes. If you currently drink every day or after work, try drinking less and making every second day an alcohol-free day. Focus on breaking your old habits and creating some new ones by drinking more calorie-free water, exercising regularly and consuming the RDIs. This will not only improve your health and reduce your waistline, but it will also increase your energy levels.

If you need to reduce your alcohol intake, don't turn to soft drinks, energy drinks or juices because these drinks contain just as much sugar and calories as the drinks you have replaced. Simple modifications in what you drink, how much and when can make a significant difference in reducing health risk factors and your ability to lose weight.

For more details refer to Stage 3: Dealing with Emotional Bonds.

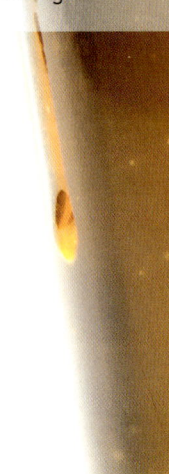

STEP 1

Meal Choices
Meal choices provides additional meal options towards obtaining one's daily recommended dietary intake. Utilize the Body Coach® Daily Food Portion Chart on page 37 to help plan your day.

Breakfast Menu

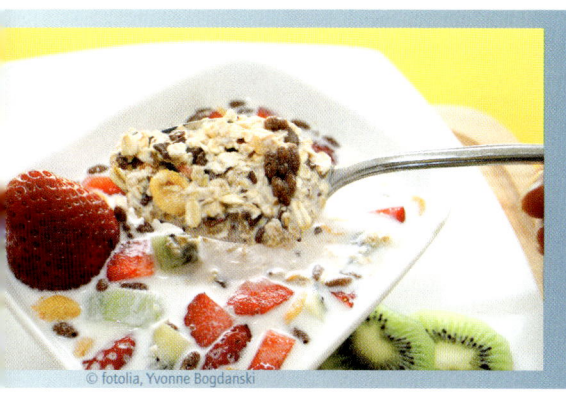

CEREAL
- 1 cup (30-40 grams) low-fat, high-fiber bran cereal (no added sugar) with 250ml low-fat milk

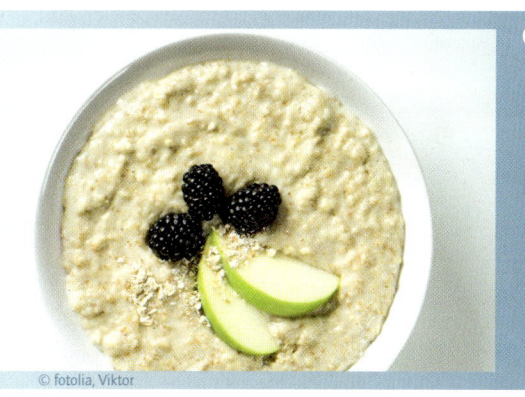

OATS
- 1 cup of oats (cooked in low-fat milk) mixed with diced banana or berries

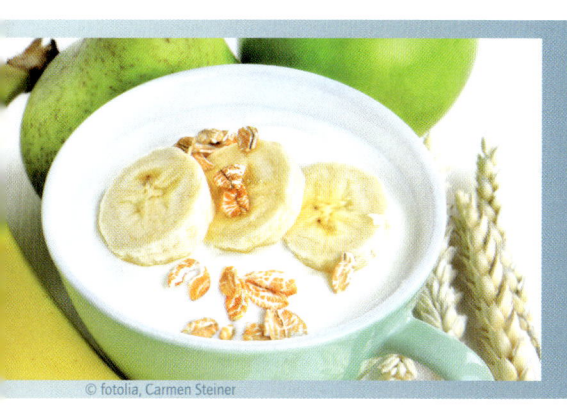

FRUIT & YOGHURT
- 1 cup of mixed diced fruit with 200 grams low-fat yogurt

WAISTLINE WORKOUT

EGGS
- 2-egg omelette filled with diced tomato, ham and bell pepper
- 2 large boiled eggs (with curry mixed) and wholegrain toast
- 2 eggs (poached, boiled or scrambled), grilled tomato on wholegrain toast
- 1 egg, grilled tomato, 1 rasher of bacon on wholegrain toast

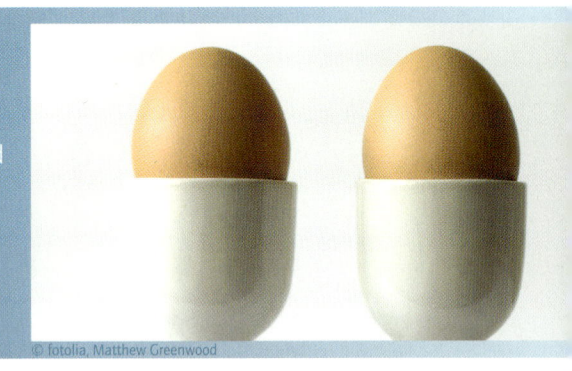

MULTIGRAIN MUFFIN
- 1 multigrain muffin, split and spread with cottage cheese and tomato
- 1 multigrain muffin split with sardines and diced tomato

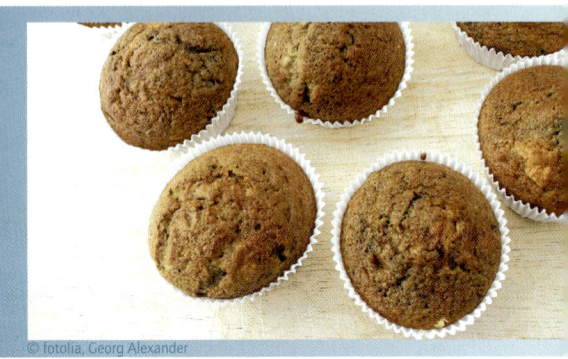

BEANS ON TOAST
- 200 grams of baked beans on wholegrain toast

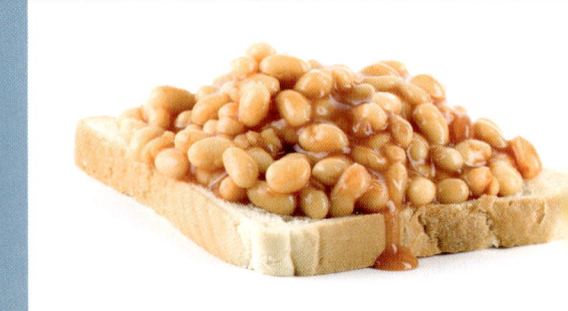

PROTEIN SMOOTHIE
- 1 glass (250ml) of low-fat milk, 2 tablespoons of low-fat natural yoghurt, 50 grams of strawberries (or mixed berries, banana, mango), 1-2 tablespoons of protein powder and ice-cubes – mixed in blender

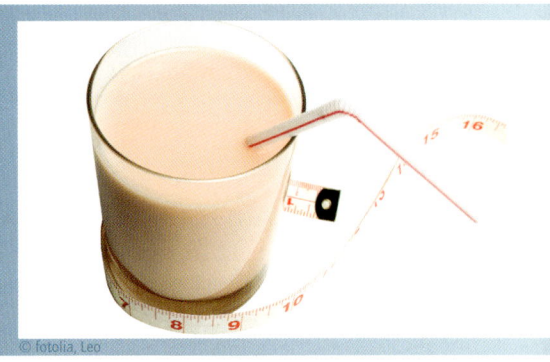

STEP 1

Snacks (mid-morning and mid-afternoon)

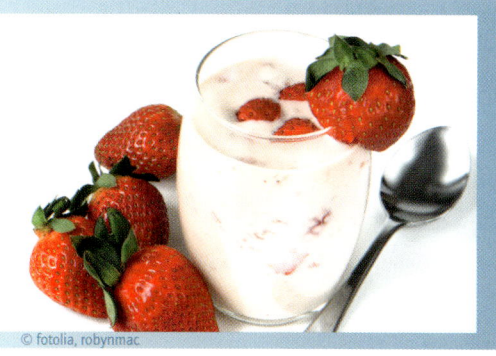

YOGHURT
- 200ml carton of low-fat yoghurt (plain or fruit) with friendly bacteria
- 200g tub of low-fat rice yoghurt

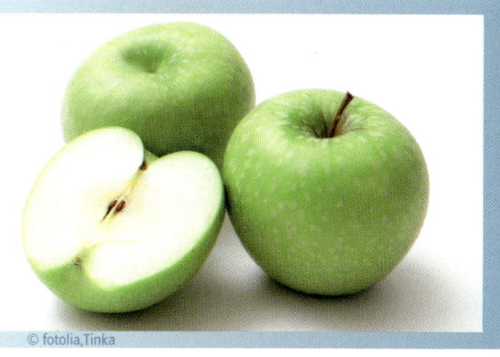

PIECE OF FRUIT
- Apple, pear, peach or kiwi fruit
- 2 apricots or plums
- 1 small banana
- 100 grams blueberries or strawberries
- Choose dried fruit such as apricots, figs, pears and peaches in small, 30g servings.

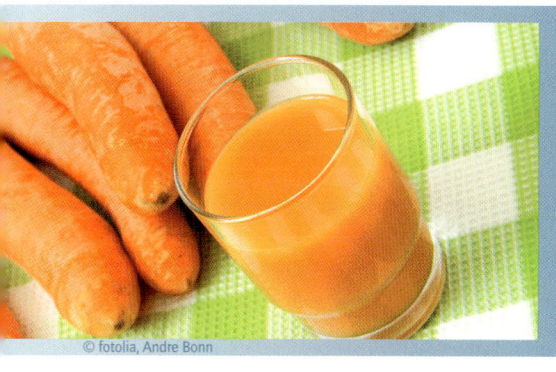

VEGETABLE JUICE
- Carrot and celery juice (add beetroot and ginger for what is known as a cleanser)

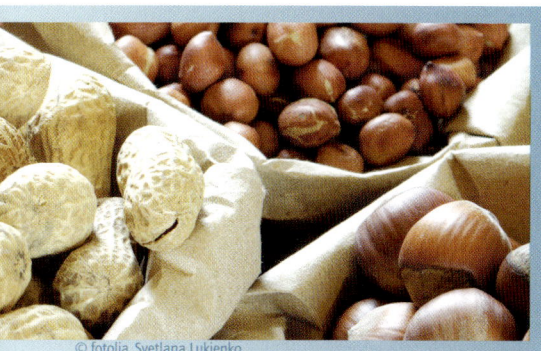

NUTS
- 1/4 cup (30 grams) of blanched or raw nuts such as: almonds, brazil nuts, walnuts

WAISTLINE WORKOUT

SNACK BARS
- 45g low-fat muesli bar
- 75g protein bar

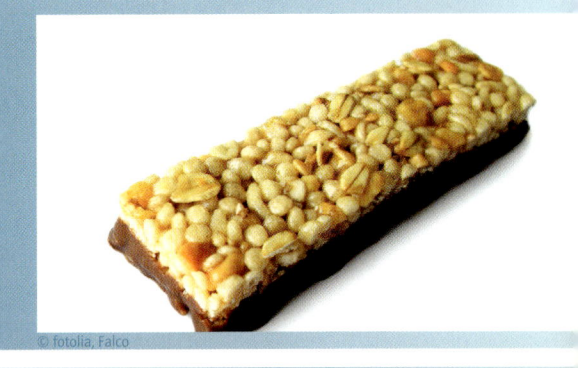

CRISPBREAD
- 1 bran crispbread with 30g slice of low-fat cheese, 20 grams of avocado and 1 slice of tomato

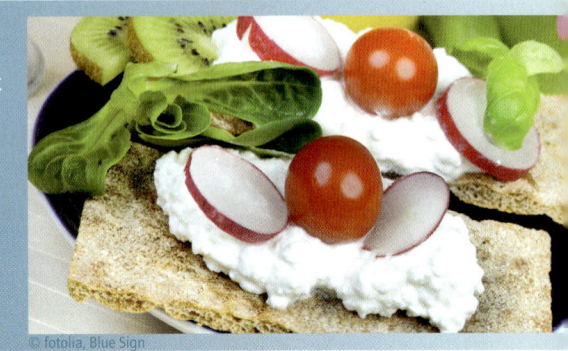

SUSHI ROLL
- 1 sushi roll – rice with protein source such as teriyaki chicken, cooked tuna, salmon or egg

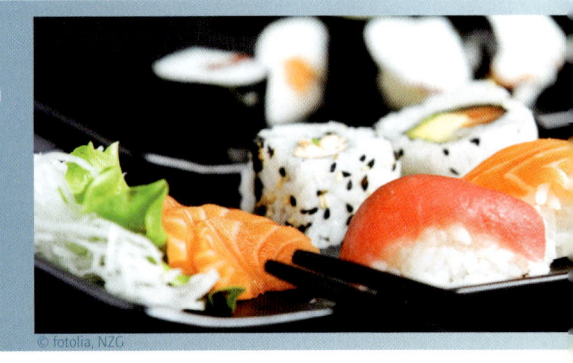

MEDICALLY APPROVED MEAL REPLACEMENT DRINK
- Meal replacement drink mixed with milk or water with appropriate vitamins and proteins and minerals

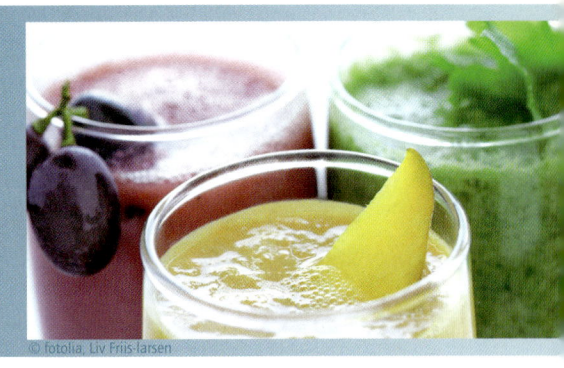

Lunch

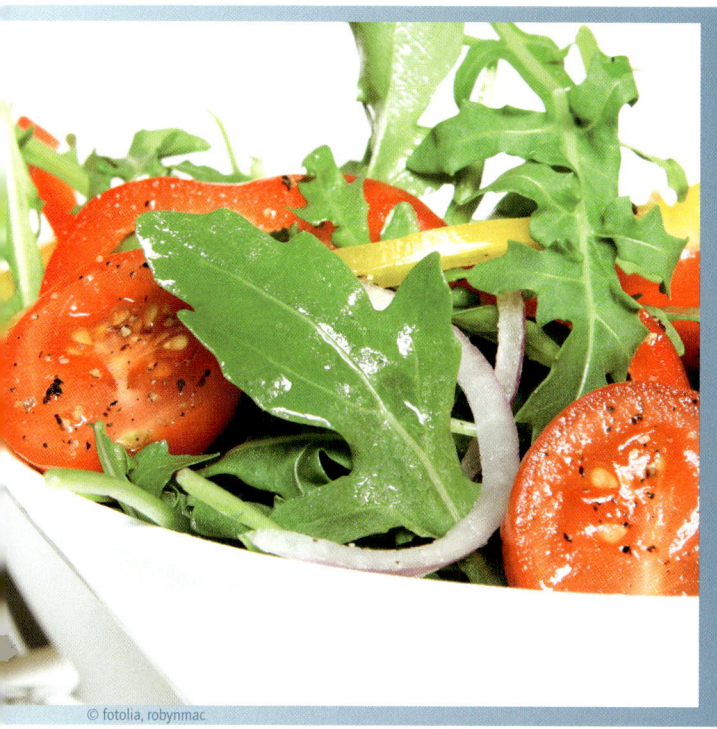

SALADS

- Protein Salad: 1 bowl of mixed color salad with 100-200 grams of lean protein, such as: chicken, lean red meat, mixed beans, grilled fish, canned fish (tuna, salmon), sardines, feta cheese, egg or mixed beans

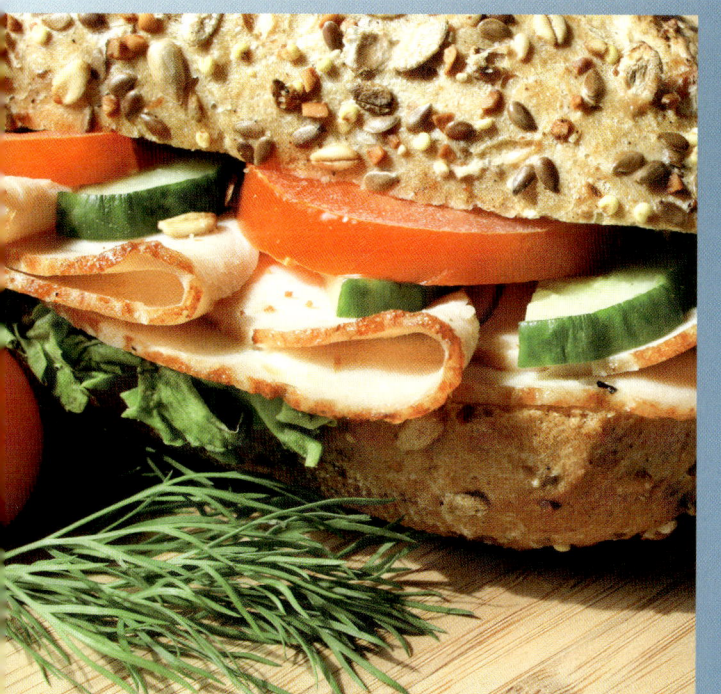

SANDWICHES

- 2 slices of wholemeal or wholegrain bread or 1 wholegrain roll or tortilla (wrap) filled with mixed salad and 100-200 grams of protein:
- lean red meat: lamb, beef, ham
- chicken or turkey
- canned fish: tuna, salmon, sardines in water
- three-bean mix
- low-fat cheese

WAISTLINE WORKOUT

SOUP
- Bowl of water-based chicken and vegetable soup
- Bowl of minestrone soup with 100 grams of lean protein source

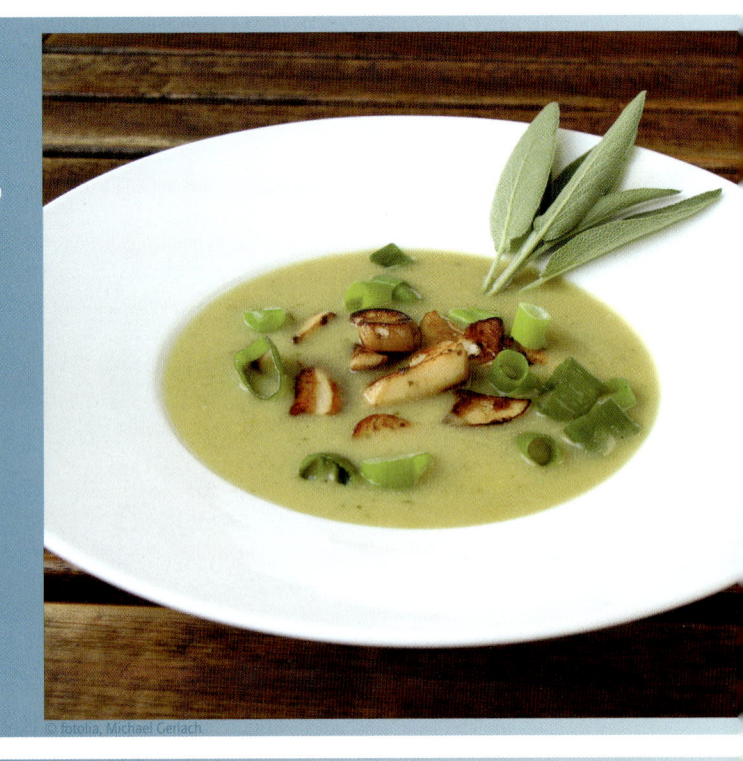

SEAFOOD
- 100-200 grams of grilled, steamed, poached or barbequed fish with fresh garden salad and oil-free dressing

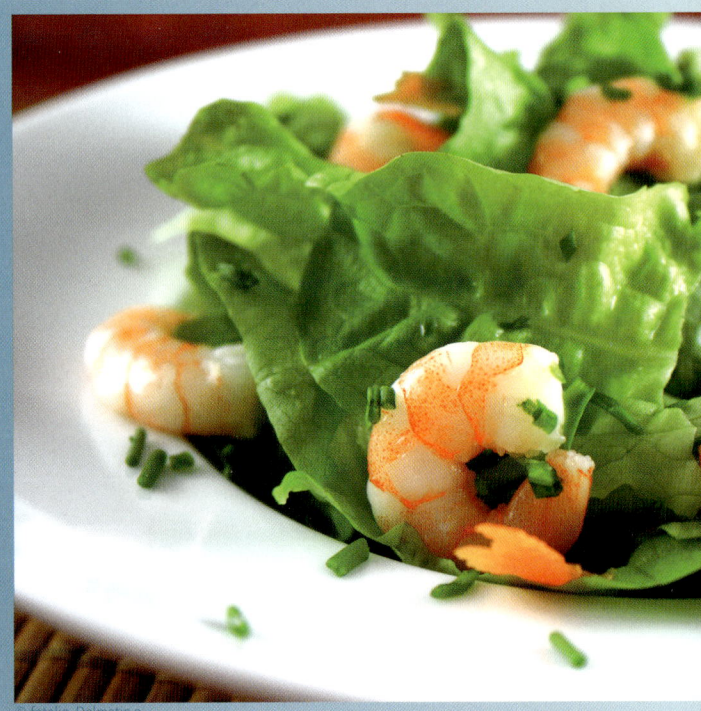

STEP 1

Dinner

SEAFOOD
- 100-200g salmon steak (barbequed or grilled) served on a bed of (100g) steamed English spinach and (100g) mashed sweet potato

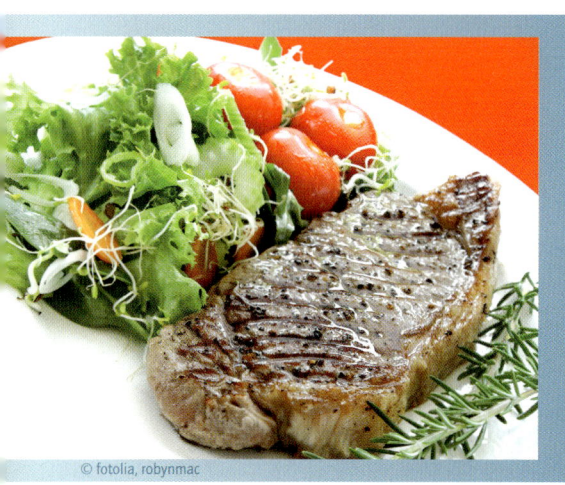

LEAN RED MEAT
- 100-200 gram sirloin steak with 40 grams of gravy, 1/2 cup of beans, sweet potato and cauliflower (no oil)
- 100-200 gram T-bone steak with 1/2 cup of mashed potato, steamed carrots and English spinach (no oil)

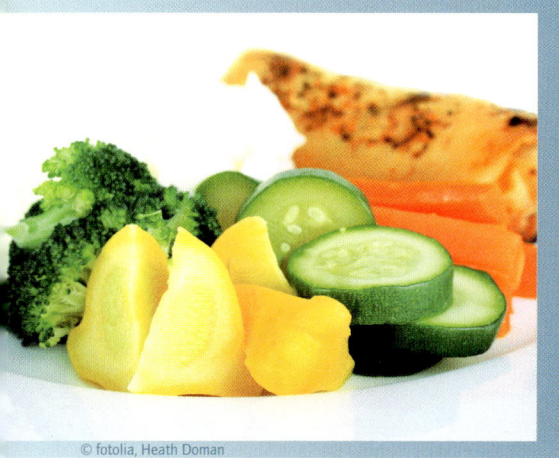

CHICKEN
- 100-200 grams chicken breast marinated in an oil-free marinade with 1/2 cup (80g) of basmati rice and 1-2 cups of mixed vegetables

WAISTLINE WORKOUT

LEAN TURKEY
- 100-200 grams of turkey breast or thigh with 50 grams of sweet and sour sauce, 1/2 cup of steamed broccoli and carrots and 1 small potato

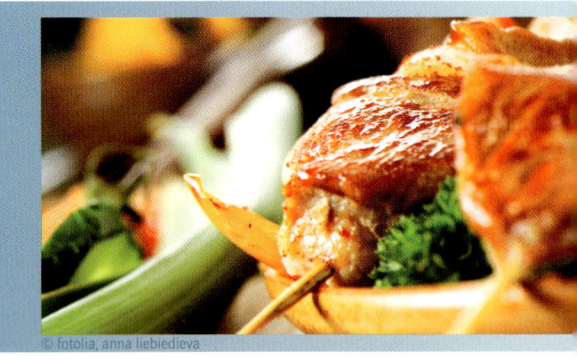

VEGETABLES
- 2 cups of mixed vegetables such as carrot, zucchini, broccoli, beans, peas and cauliflower with 100-200 grams portion of: chicken breast pieces (skin removed), lean beef, turkey or veal strips, or tofu

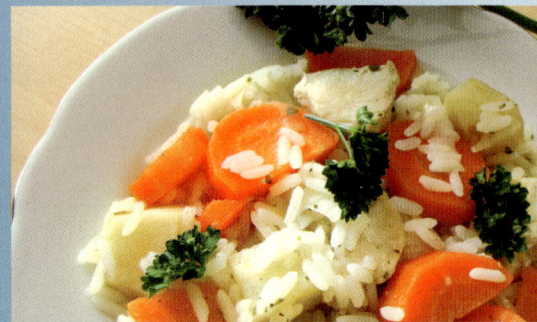

SOUP
- Bowl of vegetable soup with 100 gram protein source (chicken, lean red meat)

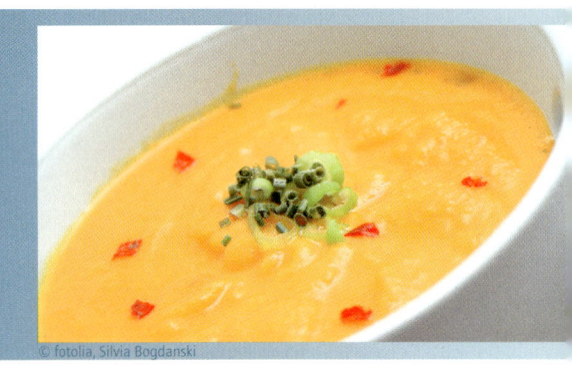

FROZEN MEALS
- A calorie-controlled frozen meal containing protein and carbohydrate source

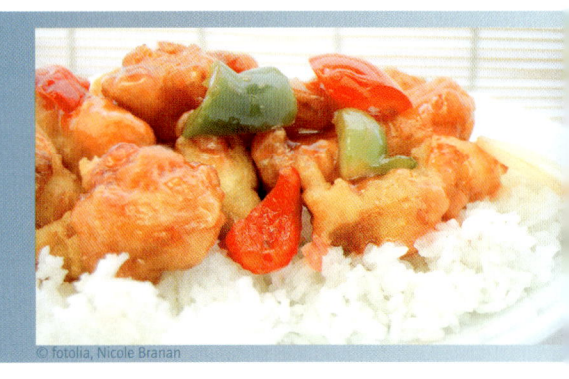

Low-Calorie Desserts

- 125 grams of low-fat custard and 100 grams of banana (diced)
- 100 grams of frozen yoghurt
- 50 grams of low-fat ice-cream and 50 grams of strawberries
- 200 gram tub of low-fat yoghurt
- 150 gram canned mixed fruits with 100g of yoghurt

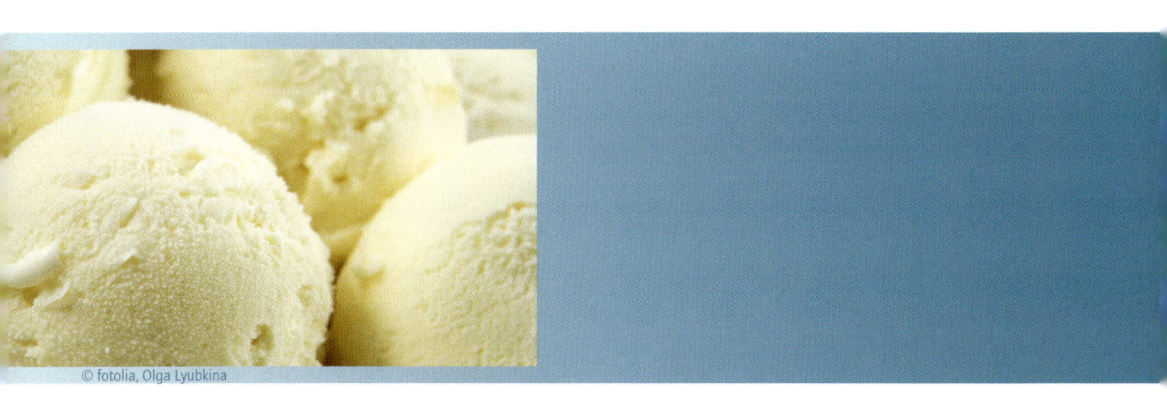

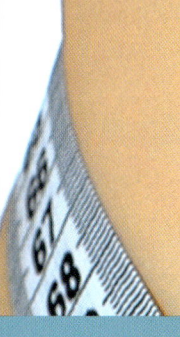

Step 2
Participating in Regular Daily Exercise

In this step you'll start with a Body Audit to establish some benchmarks followed by an exercise model for participating in regular daily exercise for muscle toning and improving heart and lung fitness.

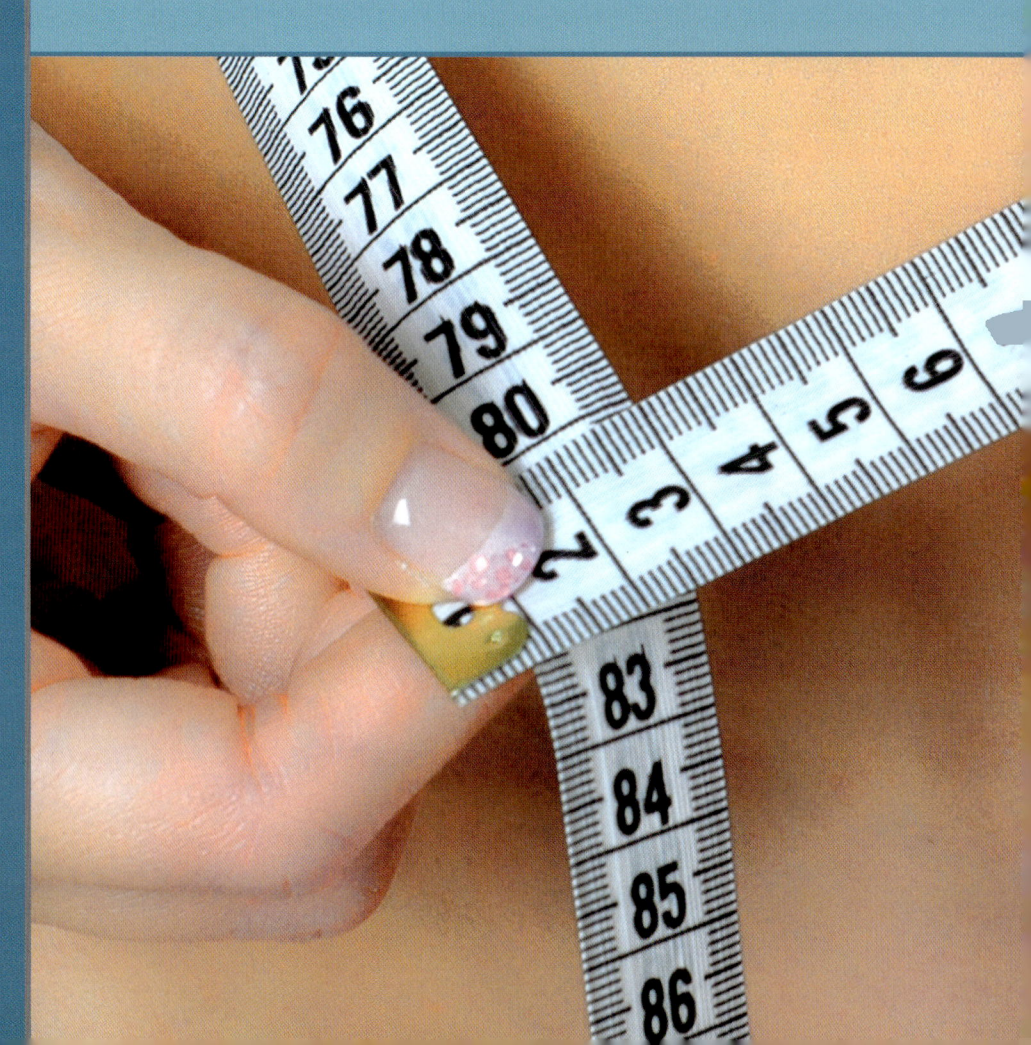

a. Body Audit

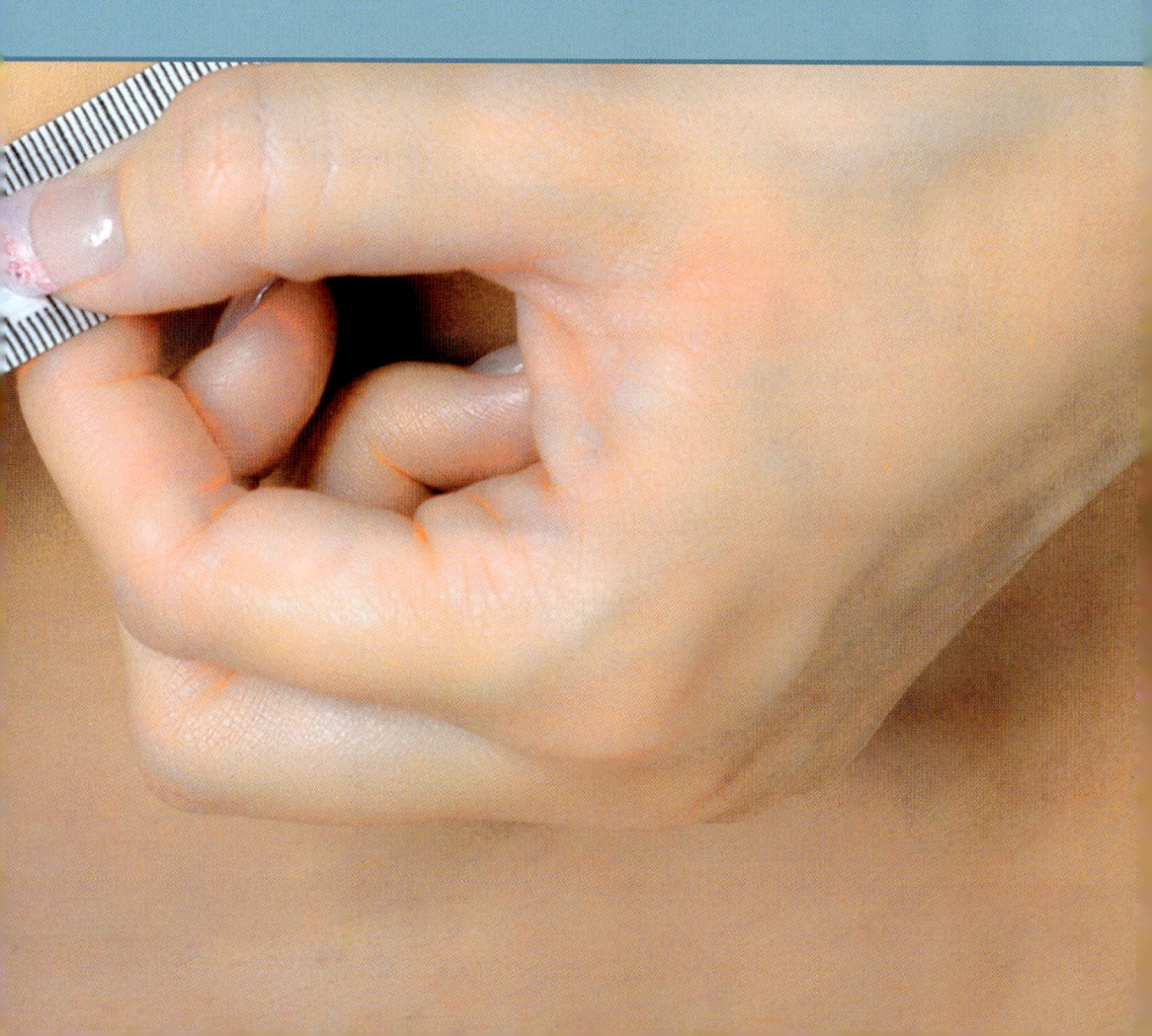

Establishing Benchmarks

Establishing a series of health benchmarks provides a blueprint of your health status. Some we can calculate, others will need to be performed by your doctor. Either way, all benchmarks are important because they act as reference points to compare with and improve upon throughout your program and in the future.

At any time, positive changes will be occurring within your body once you get started with the WW plan. By knowing your starting point and comparing these variables regularly against the recommended health standards, you will be able to establish a series of short and long term goals that will keep you motivated. The reality is that this will become a major turning point in your life as you learn how to focus on a number of important elements that ultimately lead to your best body ever.

By focusing on regular exercise, healthy eating and positive lifestyle changes, the following benchmarks can be used to gauge your success. One of your motivational goals is to lower or improve on at least one or, if necessary, all eight of these benchmark measurements throughout your 12-week journey.

1. **Body Weight**
2. **Body Mass Index (BMI)**
3. **Healthy Weight Range**
4. **Body Measurements**
5. **Photographs**
6. **Blood Pressure**
7. **Preliminary Blood Tests**
8. **Setting Goals**

STEP 2

1. Body Weight

The initial weigh in may seem daunting, but it sets a point of reference from which calculations and comparisons can be made against various health standards. These guidelines enable us to establish measurable goals to work from. In saying this, weight loss is the outcome of applying all the right ingredients, including more daily movement, regular planned exercise (fitness and strength), making healthy meal choices, meeting the recommended dietary intake, controlling meal portions, consuming more water, modifying poor habits, improving various lifestyle habits and the finer details that come from putting these into practice. When these are in balance within the body's internal structures and the mind, successful weight loss occurs. It's a good idea to use the same scales throughout wearing little or no clothing. Your weight is then used in benchmarks 2 and 3 below.

My Starting weight is = _____ kilograms (kg) or pounds (lbs)

Benchmark Test Date: _____/_____/_____

2. Body Mass Index (BMI)

One common method of determining whether you are within a healthy weight range for your height or are overweight or obese is known as the Body Mass Index or BMI. A healthy range is regarded as a BMI between 20–24.9. If you are between 25–29.9 on this scale you are considered overweight and above 30 you are considered obese. In general, the higher a person's BMI is above 25, the greater their weight-related health risks. BMI is calculated by dividing your weight in kilograms by your height in meters squared. Workout according to where you belong:

- BMI = weight in kilograms divided by height in meters squared

Example: To establish kilograms from pounds, divide total by 2.2. For example; Julie weighs 198 pounds (198 divided by 2.2 = 90 kilograms) and is 1.65 meters tall.

Her BMI is calculated as the following:

$$BMI = \frac{Weight\ (kg)}{Height\ (m) \times Height\ (m)}$$

- 90 divided by 1.65 squared (1.65 x 1.65 or 2.7225) = BMI of 33.05

Condition	BMI Scale
Underweight	below 20
Normal weight	20–24.9
Overweight	25.0–29.9
Obesity	Above 30

WAISTLINE WORKOUT

Please note: BMI does not take into account whether weight comes from fat or muscle. As a result it can overestimate people with a muscular build. This is one of the reasons a multiple array of benchmarks are used in the WW program.

Calculating your BMI   Benchmark Test Date: _____/_____/_____

Weight in kilograms _____ divided by _____ (height in meters squared) = BMI score of _____

3. Healthy Weight Range

The healthy weight range tells you about your weight relative to your height and is calculated using the BMI format between 20 and 25. The range has been worked out from studies that show people whose weight falls within this range are at less risk of medical problems. It is calculated from the BMI scale and shows you the range in weight. Work across from your height to see where you stand in relation to your weight. The difference of where you stand today and the healthy weight range should provide the long-term incentive to improve your eating habits and lifestyle.

Height			Healthy range BMI of 20		Healthy range BMI of 25	
Feet & Inches	cm		Pounds (lbs)	Kilograms (kg)	Pounds (lbs)	Kilograms (kg)
5'0"	152		100	46	124	58
5'1"	155		104	48	129	60
5'2"	157		108	50	134	62
5'3"	160		112	51	139	64
5'4"	163		116	53	144	66
5'5"	165		120	55	149	68
5'6"	167		124	56	154	70
5'7"	170		127	58	159	72
5'8"	172		131	60	164	75
5'9"	175		135	61	169	77
5'10"	177		139	63	174	79
5'11"	180		143	65	179	81
6'0"	183		147	66	184	83

Record your health weight range for your height here:

_____ to _____   Benchmark Test Date: _____/_____/_____

STEP 2

4. Body Measurements

Body measurements help gauge changes in body symmetry that weight loss cannot. Losing centimeters from around different body sites also provides ongoing motivation especially at times when your weight may plateau. Excess fat in the abdomen (stomach region) poses a greater health risk in terms of heart disease, high blood pressure and diabetes than excess fat in the hip and thigh region. The National Heart Foundation recommends, that for good health, a women's goal waist circumference should be below 80cm (and 90cm for men). Measuring different areas of the body allows you to gauge your overall body composition and the total sum of success. To record your measurements you'll need a measuring tape and a pen.

Benchmark Test Date: _____/_____/_____

Muscle	Location	Measurement in centimeters (cm) or millimeters (mm)
1. Left Arm	Measure mid point between elbow and shoulder	
2. Right Arm	Measure mid point between elbow and shoulder	
3. Waistline	Measure around naval (belly button)	
4. Hip	Measure around widest region of the hip and buttock	
5. Left Thigh	Measure the midpoint between the groin and knee	
6. Right Thigh	Measure the midpoint between the groin and knee	
7. Left Calf	Measure the widest region of the lower leg	
8. Right Calf	Measure the widest region of the lower leg	

As the body aims to regain balance in the initial phases of the program, don't be discouraged if some measurements do not change as the body is constantly changing and needs time to adjust. Instead, focus on the overall sum of total measurements in centimeters or millimeters and compare the overall difference each month. Weekly body measurements can be recorded on the WW Progress Chart on page 132.

5. Photographs

WW focuses on trimming the waistline and there's no better indicator of visual success than a photograph. Maintaining an up-to-date record of your progress by taking pictures of yourself each week provides a unique angle for comparison. Seeing your body shape change, even if you haven't lost weight, is a great way to stay motivated. Many people now have digital cameras that can be store photos on a disc or computer for easy access and comparison. Have a friend or family member take the three photographs from head to toes facing:

1. Forwards
2. Sideways
3. Backwards

Follow this by taking another three photos in the same position but from head to mid-thigh. It's a good idea to use the same setting, clothing (underwear/swimwear), stance and distance from camera for your progress photos so you can compare body shape improvements over time. You'll be amazed.

6. Blood Pressure

Blood pressure is the pressure in your arteries as your heart is pumping blood around your body. If your blood pressure is too high or too low, you increase the risk of heart failure, whereas normal blood pressure helps reduce the risks of heart attack, heart disease, stroke and kidney failure. You should always know your blood pressure level and what it means for your health.

Normal blood pressure is around 130/85. Visit your doctor for details and always follow their recommendations. See page 131 for charting your progress.

Blood Pressure Benchmark Test Date: _____/_____/_____

Doctors name: _____
Blood pressure is: _____

7. Preliminary Blood Tests

Booking a doctor's appointment for a preliminary blood test is important for anyone overweight. At the same time you have your blood pressure checked you can also ask your doctor for approval to start exercising as well taking a sample of your blood for a report on the following areas (plus any others they see appropriate):

- Cardiovascular (Cholesterol)
- Diabetes risk (Blood glucose)
- Anaemia (Haemoglobin)
- A liver function test (GGT)
- A kidney function test (Creatinine)

From this report, your doctor will provide you with the appropriate recommendations for any areas that may require improvement. Record your Preliminary Blood Test Scores below.

Blood Test Scores	Preliminary Test Results Date:
Cardiovascular (Cholesterol)	
Diabetes risk (Blood glucose)	
Anaemia (Haemoglobin)	
A liver function test (GGT)	
A kidney function test (Creatinine)	
Other test score:	

8. Setting Goals

Comparing yourself against the various health recommendations above provides a good road map in relation to where you stand today (in terms of your health) and where you need to head towards in the future. Each day you face many choices that influence your health. The way we eat and exercise is a habit that we need to turn around. Improving your eating habits and moving around more often are two major choices that contribute to positive health gains. Establishing goals in this stage helps contribute to the decisions you make. Simply knowing your blood pressure or cholesterol is high is a trigger for change, because your health is a high priority.

Weighing all these benchmarks up will help you define your health status and motivate you to continue with the program. Don't expect miracles to happen overnight, as it takes effort on your behalf. If you take it on as a challenge for improvement, your whole focus will shift from weight loss to one of thinking about your health and well-being. By caring about your health and getting in good shape, weight loss will be an extra bonus. If you really want it, you can achieve your goal. I challenge you to make a difference and show the world you can do it. Your goals and motivational drive from these benchmarks can therefore be based on one or a combination of the following:

Good Health Examples:
- Reducing your BMI below 25
- Reducing your waistline below 80cm
- Reducing your overall body composition (in centimeters or millimeters)
- Improving your blood pressure and various blood test scores performed by your doctor.

Now its time to establish your own personal goals. This can include the examples mentioned above as well as a special event or occasion you would like to look good for, such as a wedding or birthday celebration. In establishing your goals you need to be very specific with your details. For instance, I will improve my daily eating habits by preparing each meal to control my food intake and maximize my health potential; I will exercise everyday without failure to ensure I get fitter and stronger; In doing this I am setting a goal of losing up to 1kg (or 2.2lbs) per week over the next 12 weeks or 12 kilograms in total and will not lose faith along the way; In 12 weeks I want to look especially good for my friend's wedding. It's up to you to expand on these and be very specific of the outcome – knowing that even if you lose just 4 kilos (pounds) in 12-weeks that you're still successful, because you are 4 kilos lighter than where you first started off.

My Personal Goals over the next 12 weeks are:

_____
_____
_____
_____
_____
_____
_____
_____
_____

After recording your goals, return to them every day and read them out loud to yourself. Even modify and improve them. Be certain to never lose sight of the bigger picture by being in control of your destiny at all times – no excuses this time!

Accountability

Visiting your doctor is the best thing you can do to get started because it will gain your attention and kick you into action. This is because you are more than likely to be re-tested by your doctor after a set period of time (i.e. 4-8 weeks). Being accountable to your doctor or friend on a regular basis, or even a family member or personal trainer, is also a great way to stay on top of things. Once establishing these benchmarks and goals, another way to stick with it is to use special events or occasions to make improvements, such as a wedding 12 weeks from now, going on a holiday or hitting the beach this summer wearing a costume for the first time in a while. You could set your goal on rewarding yourself at the end of 12 weeks with a special gift for yourself such as buying yourself a new outfit, one you've always wanted. The various charts you will find within this book allow you to be accountable to yourself and maintain control.

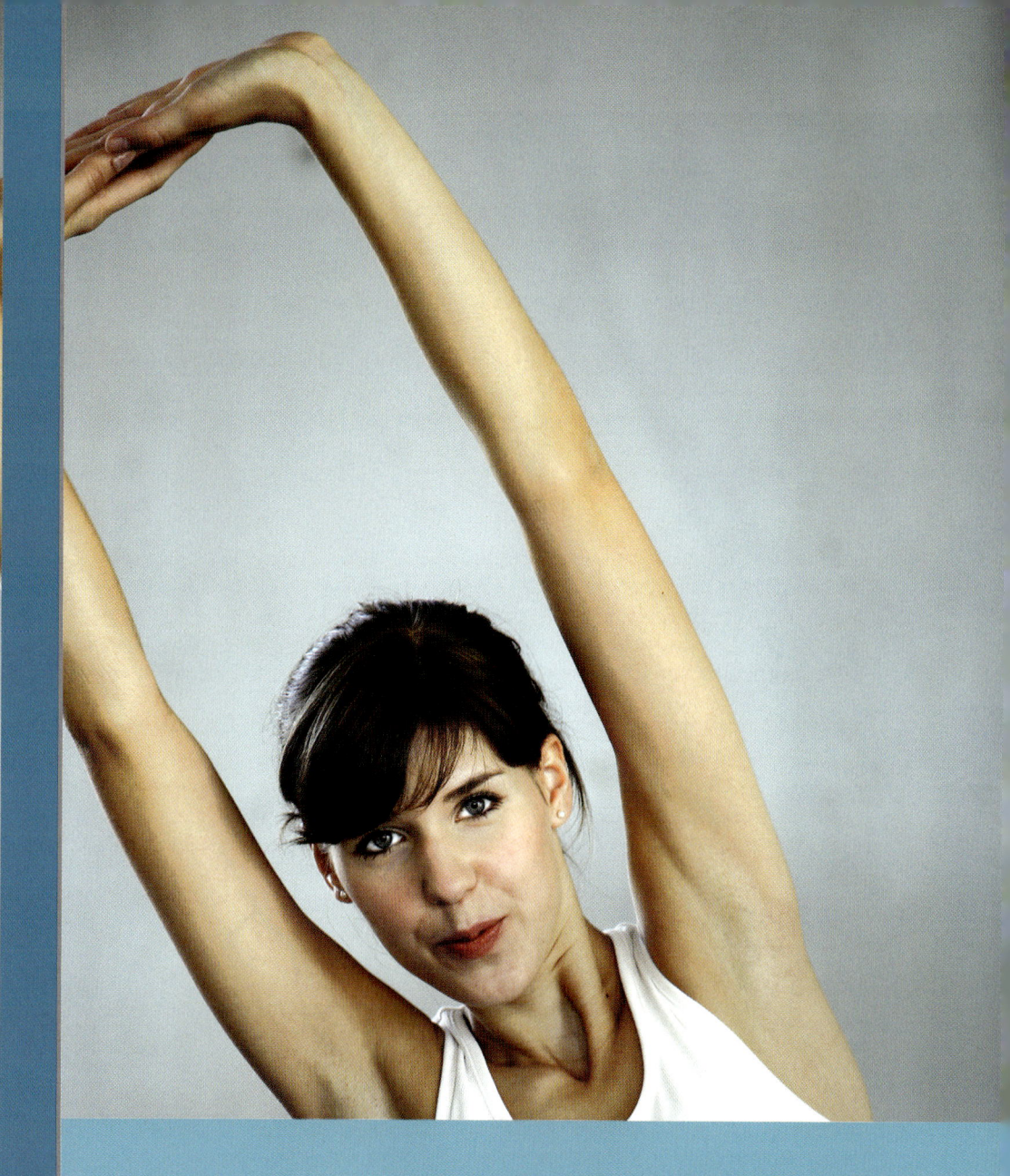

b. Exercise Plan

Phase 1: Strength Training
Phase 2: Heart and Lung Fitness

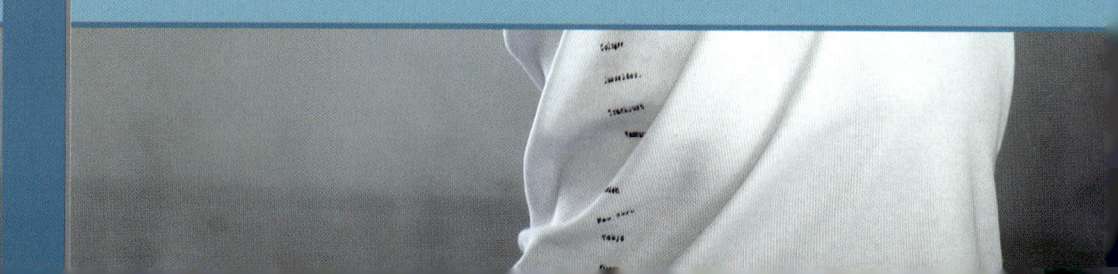

Exercise and You

Regular exercise trains your body to work more efficiently. It also helps increase your metabolic rate – *the speed at which your body uses up food as energy* – and promotes fat loss. By combining a healthy eating plan with regular exercise, you have the perfect ingredient to build your sexiest body ever.

Exercise specifically involves planned physical activity with a specific objective such as improving your cardiovascular (heart and lung) fitness, strengthening and toning your muscles, and the end outcomes of reshaping your body and losing weight. The unique approach of the WW Exercise Plan is designed with all these in mind.

WW in Action

Rapid weight loss, quick fix diets and restrictive eating all lead to one thing – a pear shaped body with larger looking thighs. The reason for this is that when the body is deprived the first thing it generally does is strip precious muscle tissue from the upper body for energy. In most cases you will lose weight from the upper body and even have a slimmer looking face, but look below and your hip and thigh region now looks even larger. It's a common mistake women make over and over again.

To help turn this around, WW includes a unique strength training and cardiovascular (heart and lung) exercise approach that helps preserve lean muscle, rev up your metabolism and target fat stores. As a result, most people gain leaner muscle and even drop down a size or two in clothing after they start the program. This is because fat is bulky and less dense and takes up twice as much space as muscle.

The WW Plan

Many people believe that when you exercise a specific body part, such as the thighs or abdominal muscles, the involved muscles burn the surrounding fat and you can reduce this area. Even those who walk or jog regularly are disappointed with lack of results they achieve. Now, I don't mean to disappoint you at this moment but spot reduction of fat from the thighs or abs does not happen without training the whole body. It is important to understand that in most cases with poor dieting habits and sporadic exercise, women will generally lose weight from the upper body first – face, neck, shoulders, chest and arms. Then when your weight loss plateaus and you give up whatever diet you're on, you often gain a few extra kilos as well as a larger looking thigh region. A term I refer to as the pear-shaped syndrome.

To turn this event around, the WW approach focuses on teaching you how to regain good overall body symmetry. The unique exercise plan that follows has you exercising to regain muscle tone of the upper body region and for a good reason. Strength training here offsets the loss in muscle mass and strength associated with normal ageing and poor dietary habits. The good news is if you already exercise (walk, jog, cycle, aerobics) you are at an advantage because it's just a simple shift towards strength training where you will achieve the results you've always been looking for. Men are at an advantage here over women here because men build muscle more easily than women due to their testosterone advantage.

So, don't worry about building bulky muscles, its harder than you think for woman. What is more likely to happen is, that your upper body region will become firmer, leaner and more toned. In the initial stages on training you may feel a 'pump up' of the muscles; this is just the blood pooling in the area being exercised to help with repair and recovery, which soon returns to normal. Just look at Karen's results in the photos on page 16 to remind yourself of the results you can achieve.

Strengthening and toning your upper body allows it to repair and rebuild leaner muscle tissue. While this is happening, the extra energy required is more likely to come from the fat stores located at the thigh region, whereas, before with poor dieting or cardiovascular exercise alone (walking, jogging, aerobics, etc.), this muscle tissue was lacking. Strengthening the abdominal, buttock and leg regions are still vital, because it is important to tighten and firm them, but the major focus for stripping fat off the abdominals and hip and thigh regions comes from strengthening both the upper body and lower body regions as I will show you in the exercise programs that follow.

In comparison, men and women are almost equal in terms of their leg strength, but when it comes to the upper body with push-ups and chin exercises, for example, there is quite a hefty difference. Most people will avoid exercises and things they can't do well. In our case, this is the line you need to step over to get the results you desire. While you may be tempted to train only the areas that need shaping, the main aspect we will be focusing on is regaining body symmetry. This means if you currently have larger thighs and hip (pear-shape body), developing your shoulders, chest, arms and back muscles can make your lower body region look smaller. Once body symmetry develops and your fitness and strength improves, your body will start to work more efficiently and a new approach is applied. Until then stick with the program at hand to regain and maintain the lean muscle tissue of the upper body because this is where the main results will come from.

Body Symmetry Strength Routine

To achieve the necessary body symmetry to overcome this 'pear-shape syndrome' or belly fat, there are two specific phases of the WW Exercise Plan:

1. **Muscle Toning Strength Training**
2. **Heart and Lung (Cardiovascular) Fitness**

Phase 1: Strength Training

Your muscles are the energy burning powerhouse of your body. The better condition they are in, the greater your body's ability is in burning more calories and fat, even whilst you are resting. Strength training itself works in a progressive manner. Initially, we will be working on gaining muscle endurance using light hand weights or performing low intensity body weight exercises over an extended period of time (ie. 30 seconds or more). This approach allows your body and its muscles and joints time to adapt. As you become stronger and more confident, the demand to increase the resistance rises. This is when the body can make changes. In the initial phase of training, finding the right exercise to suit your level of strength and ability is important. Undergoing a physical assessment by a qualified health professional such as a physiotherapist will help determine the best starting point for you.

Ultimately, the key to effective body changes is when strength exercises start to fatigue muscles at around 8 repetitions (reps) and before 12 (reps). This can be achieved in a number of ways:

- In body weight exercises increasing the lever length, for example, moving from a kneeling push-up to performing push-ups on the hands and toes – increases the demand of the exercise and holding correct body alignment (or posture).
- In strength training, for example lifting free weight (hand weights, dumbbells or barbells) or using weight training machines, it involves increasing the resistance or amount of weight being lifted and the demand on the body where changes occur.
- Alternatively, slowing each repetition of the exercise down to increase the time the muscle is under tension can help make easier exercises become harder. For example, 10 push-ups could easily be performed in 10 seconds if you were fit (ie. 1 second per rep x 10 reps = 10 seconds). Yet, by slowing the exercise down and performing one repetition every 3 seconds increases the time the muscle is being held under tension (ie. 3 seconds per rep x 10 reps = 30 seconds) and greater results will occur. In saying this, once an exercise becomes easy you can change the type of exercise being performed for the same muscle group.

You can also perform a different exercise that targets the same muscle group. For example, a chin-up exercise using your own body weight and a Lat Pull-down exercise using a weight, target the same muscle group.

Exercise Terminology

Before you get started there are a few key exercise terms you'll need to understand:

- **Repetition** = One execution of an exercise (i.e. up and down in a push-up).
- **Set** = A series of repetitions (i.e. 10 reps = 1 set). You may be asked to perform 3 sets of 10 reps.
- **Recovery** = Time for muscles to recover after a set before repeating (i.e. 30 seconds rest).
- **Time under tension** = The speed at which you perform each repetition (i.e. 2 seconds lowering, 2 seconds raising).

- **Circuit Training** = A form of muscle endurance training using a light load that works one muscle group (exercise) for a set period (ie. 30 seconds) and then moves onto another muscle group (exercise) with minimal rest in-between.
- **Strength Training** = Using a resistance such as body weight, hand weights or weight machines to improve muscle strength and tone.
- **Warm-up** = Spending several minutes before training performing light movements that raise a light sweat to increase body temperature and your heart rate for the physical demands that lie ahead.
- **Stretching** = Holding a muscle in a position for a set period of time (i.e. 15 seconds) to help reduce muscular tension, increases range of movement, pliability and flexibility. Stretching can be performed after warming up the body and during training. It is most beneficial after completing a training session.

3B's Principle™: Pre-Exercise Set-up

Every exercise has a number of key elements to consider when setting up and performing a movement. Applying correct technique from the onset will help establish good form which is ultimately maintained until the repetitions or set is completed. After reviewing Anatomy of Movement, the key elements required in order to maintain good body position whilst exercising form part of a simple exercise set-up phrase I've termed the **3B's Principle™**:

1. Brace
Activating and bracing your abdominal muscles whilst exercising is important because it helps increase awareness of your body position as well as helping unload any stress placed on the lower back region.

2. Breath
In foundation and core-strength training, you **breathe-out** when you exert a force – such as pushing the bar up and extending the arms in the bench press exercise or rising up straight from a squat position. You then **breathe-in** with recovery – such as lower the bar towards the chest with the bench press exercise or lowering the body and bending the legs when performing a squat. Breathing should remain constant throughout each exercise.

3. Body Position
To complete the 3B's Principle™, the third B relates to one's ability to hold a good body position and technique with each exercise. In all exercises, ensure good head and neck, spine and pelvic alignment is maintained at all times with the rest of the body. The overall focus of each exercise should therefore be on quality of the movement.

So, next time you perform any exercise, simply apply the 3B's Principle™ from start to finish in order maintain correct technique and body posture to help maximize strength gains.

Muscle Toning Strength Training - Routine 1

Using your own body weight is a great way to get started with toning and reshaping your body. These exercises can be performed anytime, anywhere and its free! There are two specific Strength Training Routines to follow. The first is for the upper body (2-3 x week) and the second is for the lower body including the stomach (abdominal) muscles (1-2 x week). Within each routine you have the option of strength training or circuit training. The key to strength training is to never exercise the same muscle group two days in a row as this allows time for muscles to tone and rebuild. As your strength builds, it's natural that the exercises, reps, sets and routines you perform will need to be modified for improvements to occur. The programs below therefore aim to get you started with the process. You may start with Routine 1 or 2 depending on your training background and lifestyle circumstances such as working out at home or being a member of the gym.

Before getting started, use the following chart to assist in your preparation.

Equipment	• Chair or bench • Hand weights
Clothing	• Wear comfortable sports clothing
Warm-up	• 3 – 5 minutes of brisk walking to gradually increase heart rate and raise a light sweat to prepare body for the exercises ahead. • Follow this with a period of stretching. Hold stretches for each muscle group for 15-30 seconds
Workout Time	• 15 minutes • Exercise to your favorite music • Exercise with a friend
Cool Down	• Allow body to return to pre-exercise state with 5-minute cool-down period followed by stretching • Remember to drink lots of water before, during and after your activity (don't wait until you feel thirsty or start sweating)
Exercise Tips	• Always see your doctor to gain approval to start any new exercise or routine • Brace stomach muscles to support spine • Always maintain good posture and body alignment by focusing on the task at hand • Maintain **deep breathing** throughout each exercise. Breath in on recovery and breath out when exerting a force. • Stop exercising if you feel unwell, have pain or have difficulty breathing. Do not start exercising again until you have talked with your doctor.

STEP 2

1. Body Coach® Upper Body Home Workout Routine

- 2-3 x week – eg. Mon, Thurs (or Mon, Wed, Fri)

Upper Body Routine	1. Strength Training – Reps, Sets & Recovery	2. Circuit Training – Muscle Endurance
1. Modified Push-ups page 71	• 3 sets of 8 – 12 reps. • Rest 30–60 seconds and then repeat set • If the exercise becomes easy, increase the resistance or slow each repetition down	• Exercise for 15-30 seconds • Move directly from one exercise to the next for all 6 exercises. • Rest one minute at the completion of all 6 exercises and then repeat circuit
2. Arm Dips page 73		
3. Arm Curls page 74		
4. Side Raises page 75		
5. Shoulder Press page 76		
6. Single Arm Row page 77	• 3 sets of 8 – 12 reps both arms. No rest – move from one arm across to the other	

Please Note: Exercise summary and illustrations on the following pages.

WAISTLINE WORKOUT

Target Muscles – Upper Body

Front Side of Body **Rear Side of Body**

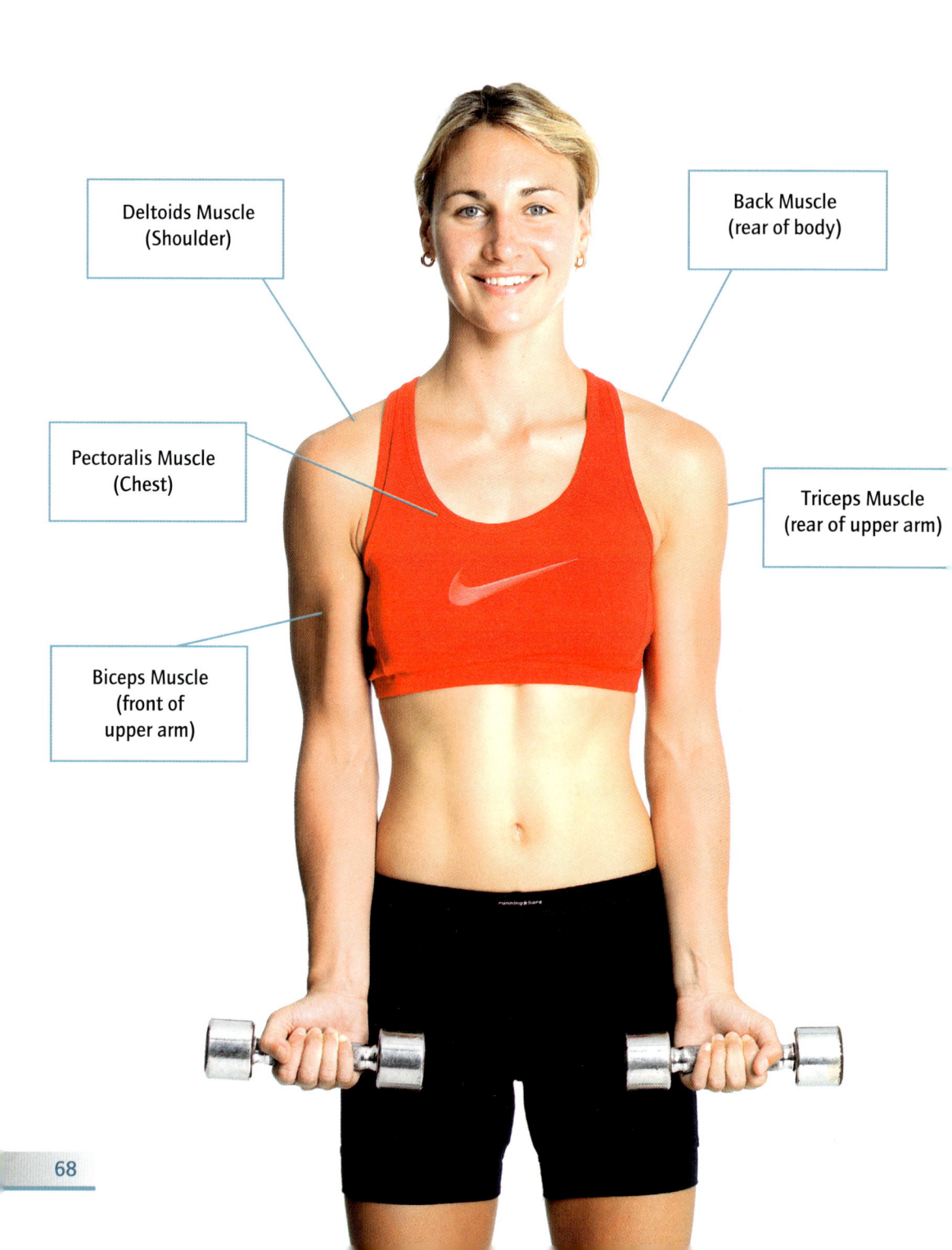

Deltoids Muscle (Shoulder)

Back Muscle (rear of body)

Pectoralis Muscle (Chest)

Triceps Muscle (rear of upper arm)

Biceps Muscle (front of upper arm)

2. Body Coach® Lower Body Home Workout Routine

- 1-2 x week – eg. Wed (or Tues, Thurs)

Lower Body Routine	1. Strength Training – Reps, Sets & Recovery	2. Circuit Training – Muscle Endurance
1. Half Squat page 78	• 3 sets of 8 – 12 reps. Rest 30 seconds	• Exercise for 15-30 seconds
2. Stationary Lunge page 79	• 3 sets of 8 – 12 reps both legs. No rest – move from one leg across to the other	• Move directly from one exercise to the next, for all 6 exercises. Rest one minute at the completion of all 6 exercises and then repeat circuit
3. Kick Backs page 80		
4. Single Leg Calf Raises page 81	• Rest 30 seconds between exercises	Note: If the exercise becomes easy, increase the resistance or slow each repetition down
5. Stomach Crunch page 82	• 3 sets of 8 – 12 reps. • Rest 30 seconds	
6. Cross-Overs page 83	• 3 sets of 8 – 12 reps both sides. No rest – move from one side across to the other	

Please Note: Exercise summary and illustrations on the following pages.

WAISTLINE WORKOUT

Target Muscles – Mid & Lower Body

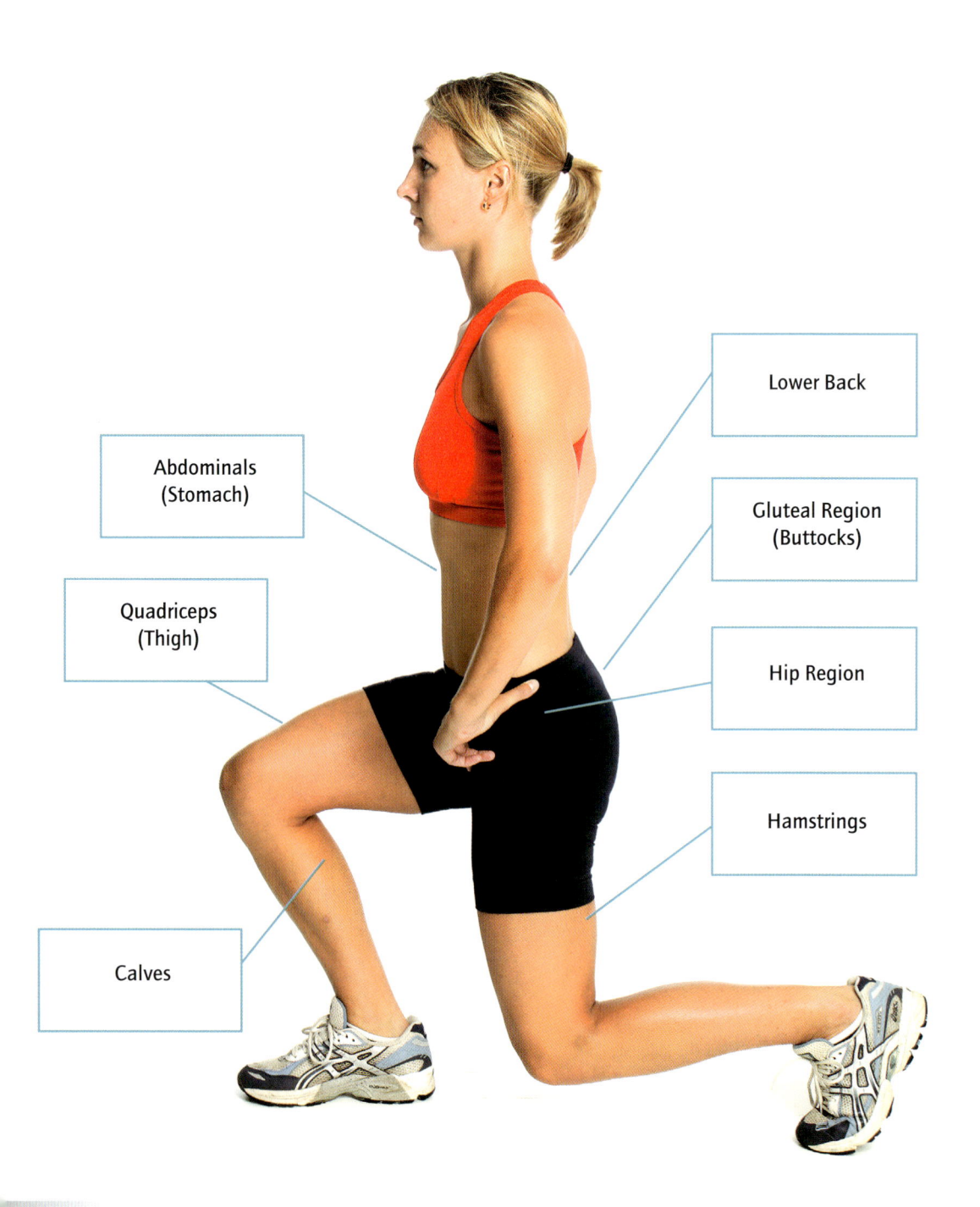

Lower Back

Abdominals (Stomach)

Gluteal Region (Buttocks)

Quadriceps (Thigh)

Hip Region

Hamstrings

Calves

Body Coach® Upper Body Home Workout Routine
1. Modified Push-ups Option (Chest & Arms)

Choose 1 exercise from below:

(1a) Chair - Kneeling: Beginner level

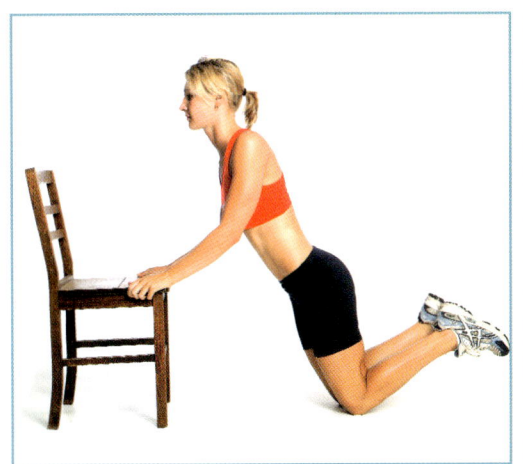

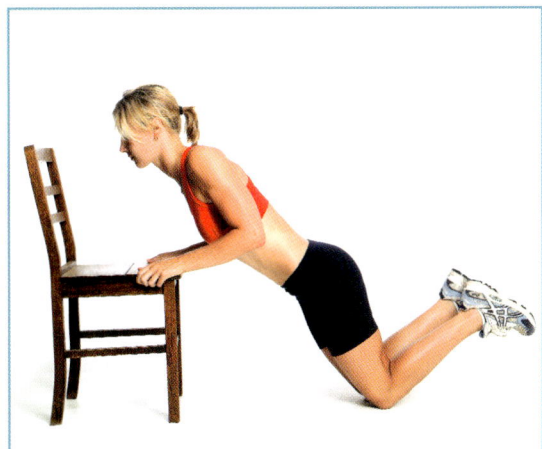

Position:
Kneel on ground in front of chair and extended arms forward onto seat. Brace stomach muscles.

Action:
Lower chest towards seat by bending the elbows, then straighten arms and raise body to starting position.

WAISTLINE WORKOUT

(1b) Kneeling – Ground: Intermediate level

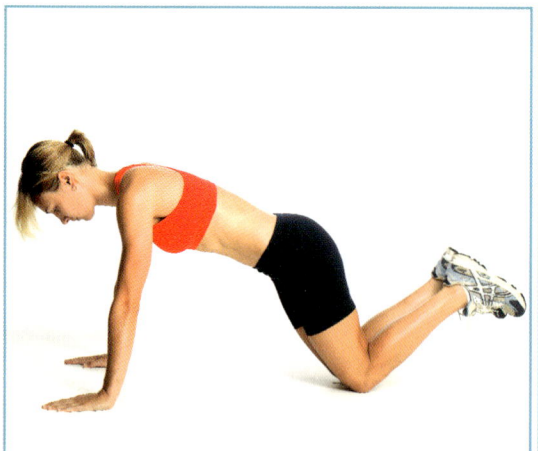

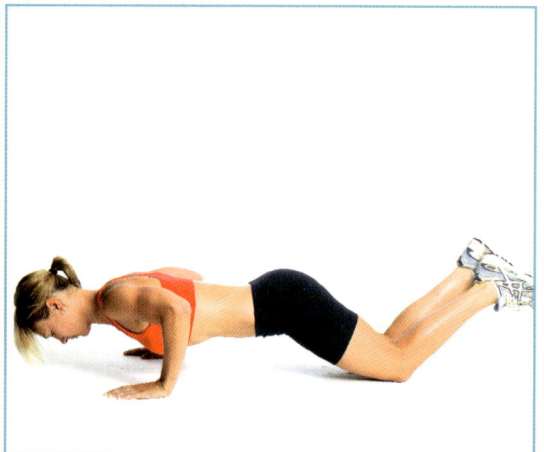

Position:
Kneel on ground with hands shoulder width apart. Lean forward so eyeline is forward of fingers. Brace stomach muscles.

Action:
Lean forwards as you lower the chest to ground in line with the hands by bending the elbows, then straighten arms and raise body to starting position. Keep elbows close to the body when lowering and raising.

Option: Perform this exercise standing at an angle with hands on solid table (or kitchen bench) or a more advanced version in a front support position on hands and feet with body kept straight.

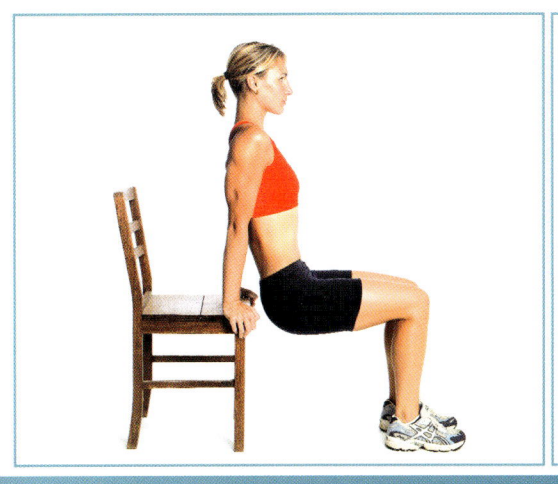

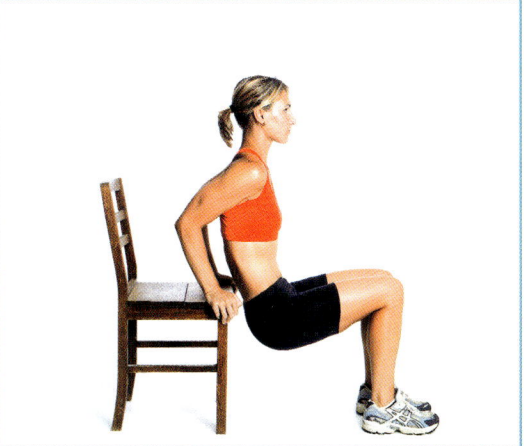

2. Arm Dips (Triceps)

Position:
Place hands on edge of solid chair or bench. Extend legs forward of the body with legs bent at 90 degrees.

Action:
Lower body by bending arms towards 90-degree angle. Then, raise body up by straightening arms.

Option: Increase intensity of exercise by extending one leg forward.

WAISTLINE WORKOUT

3. Arm Curls (Biceps)

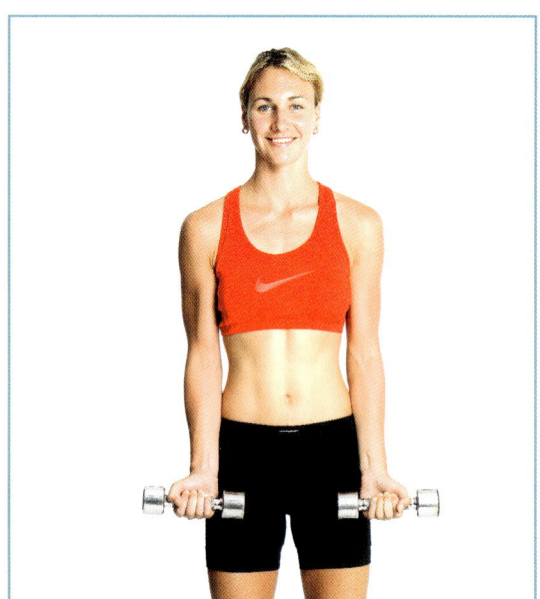

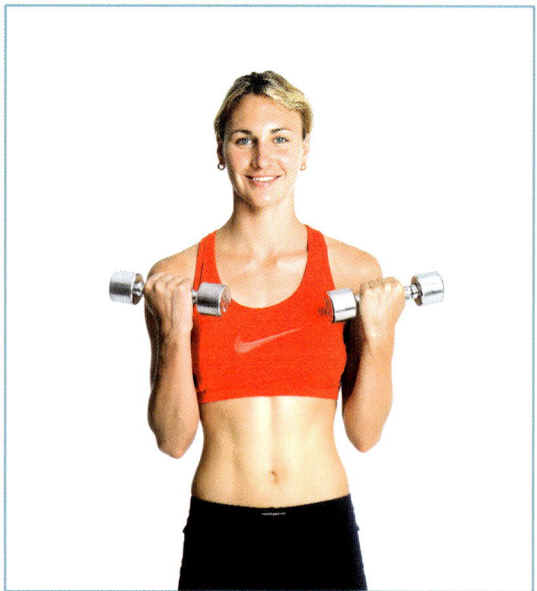

Position:
Standing with feet shoulder width apart, grip hand weights close to the side of the body with palms facing forwards.

Action:
Bend elbows and raise hands to shoulders, then lower and straighten arms.

4. Side Raises (Shoulders)

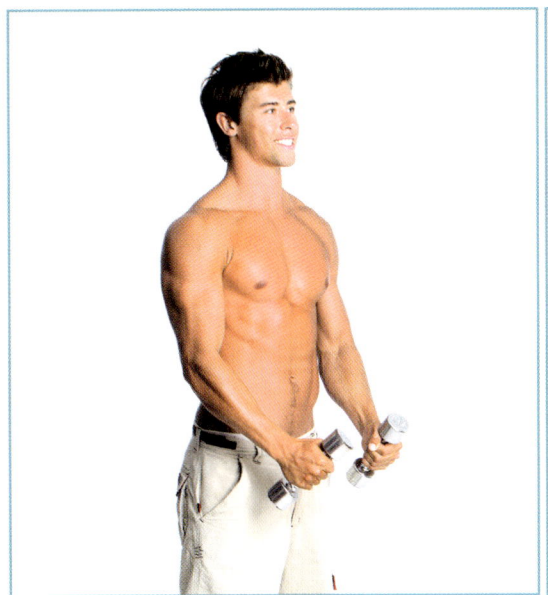

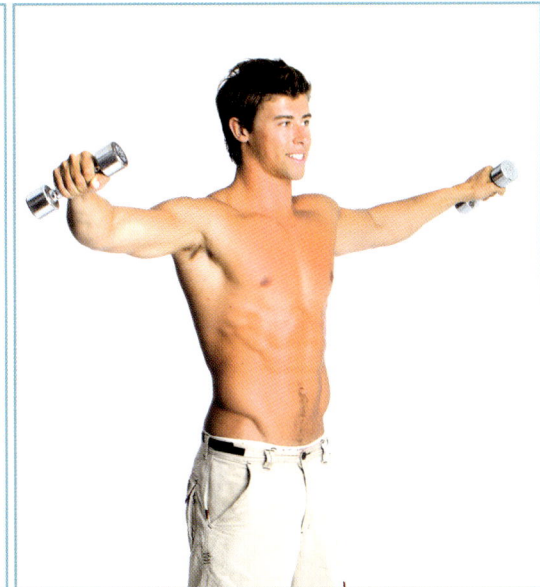

Position:
Standing with feet shoulder width apart, grip hand weights with palms together in front of the body. Brace stomach muscles.

Action:
Raise arms up to side, parallel to ground, and then lower. Repeat with opposite arm.

Option: Bend arms and raise elbows up to side.

WAISTLINE WORKOUT

5. Shoulder Press (Shoulders)

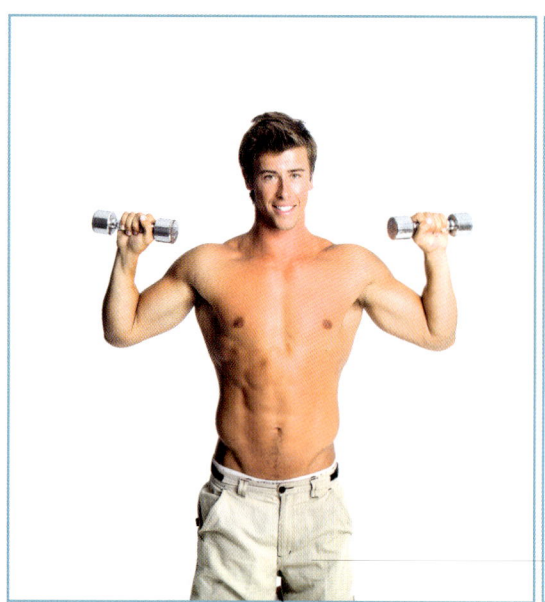

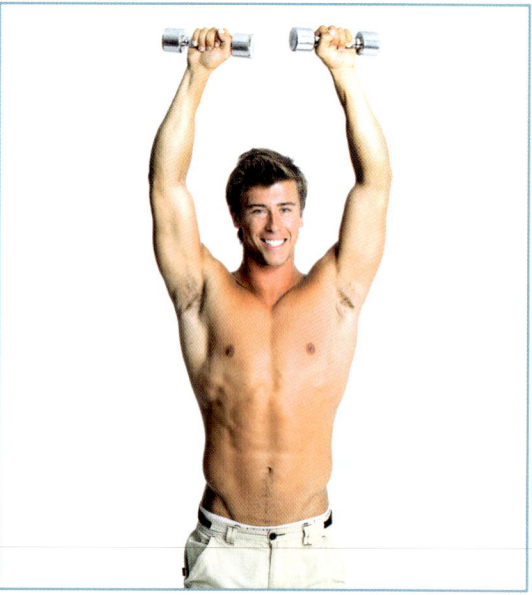

Position:
Standing with feet shoulder width apart, grip hand weights at shoulder level. Brace stomach muscles.

Action:
Push arms up overhead without arching lower back, then lower.

Option: Start with elbows and hands closer together in front of the body and push overhead.

STEP 2

6. Single Arm Row (Back)

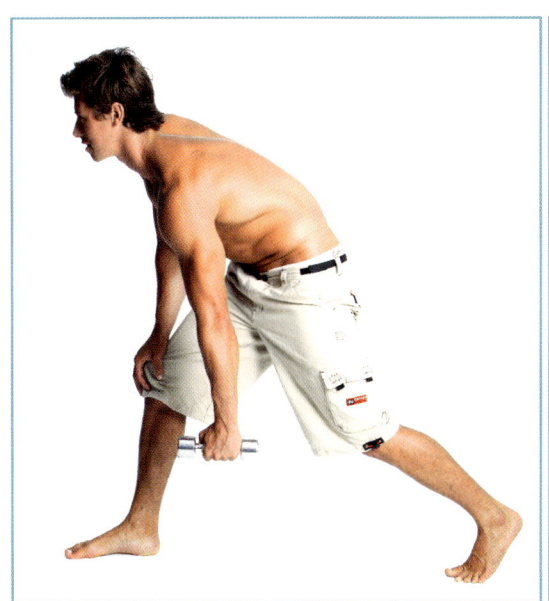

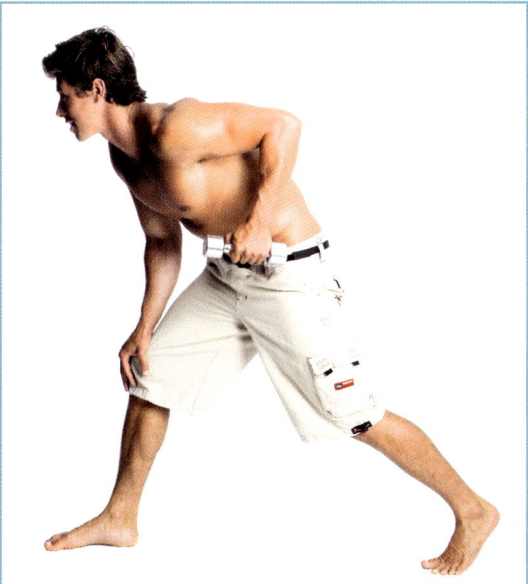

Position:
Standing in a forward lunge position, with hand resting on forward knee and the outside hand holding hand weight.

Action:
Raise arms up to side of body until upper arm is parallel to ground, then lower. Repeat with opposite arm.

Option: Place one hand on chair for support

Body Coach® Lower Body Home Workout Routine

1. Half-Squat (Legs and Buttocks)

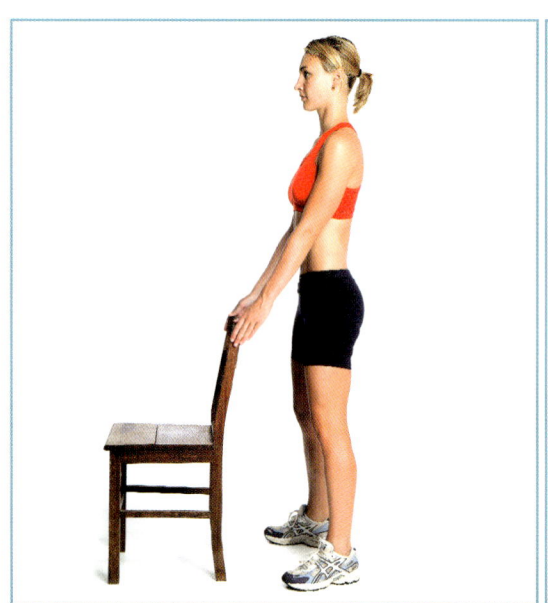

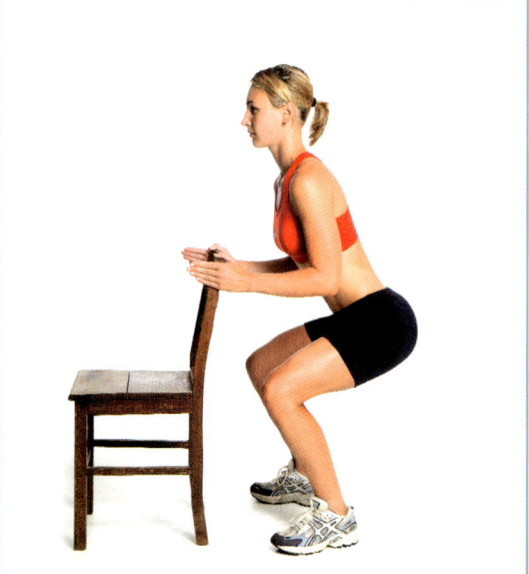

Position:
Stand with feet shoulder-width apart behind chair. Place hands on chair for support if required, otherwise extend the arms forward parallel to ground.

Action:
Lower body by pushing buttocks backwards and bending at the knees towards a 90-degree angle and then raise body up by straightening legs.

Note: When pushing buttocks backwards, ensure feet are always flat on the ground and knees follow alignment of toes (foot angle).

2. Stationary Lunge (Buttocks and Legs)

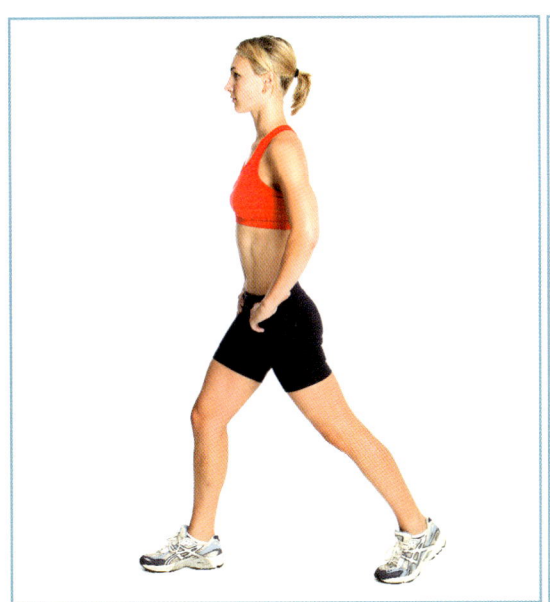

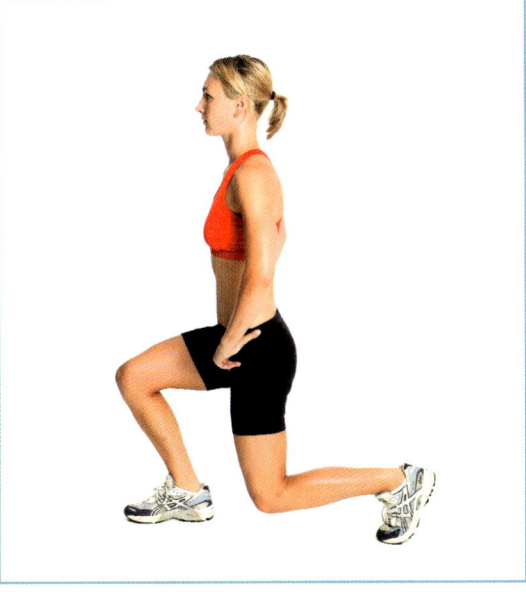

Position:
Place hands on hips and extend one leg forward into lunge position.

Action:
Lower body by bending both knees simultaneously and lowering rear knee towards floor, then returning to the upright position. Repeat with opposite leg.

WAISTLINE WORKOUT

3. Kick Backs (Hip & Buttocks)

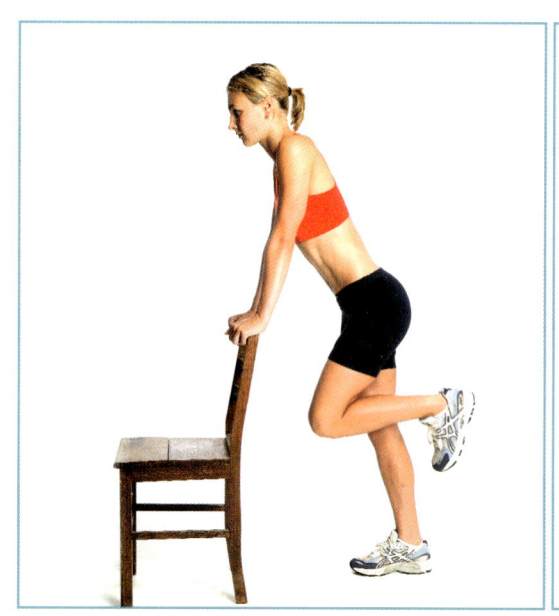

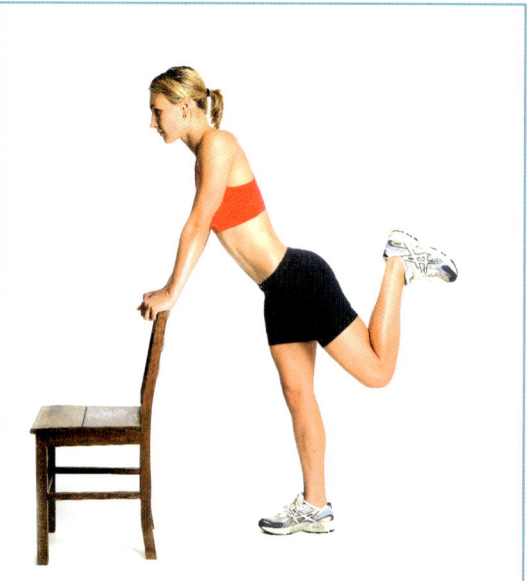

Position:
Rest hands on rear of chair, bend one leg and raise foot off ground. Lean body slightly forward from waist and brace stomach muscles.

Action:
Keeping hips square, pulse foot upwards and down over short distance – avoid any low back arching or twisting leg out. Repeat with opposite leg.

4. Single Leg Calf Raises (Balance & Calf Muscles)

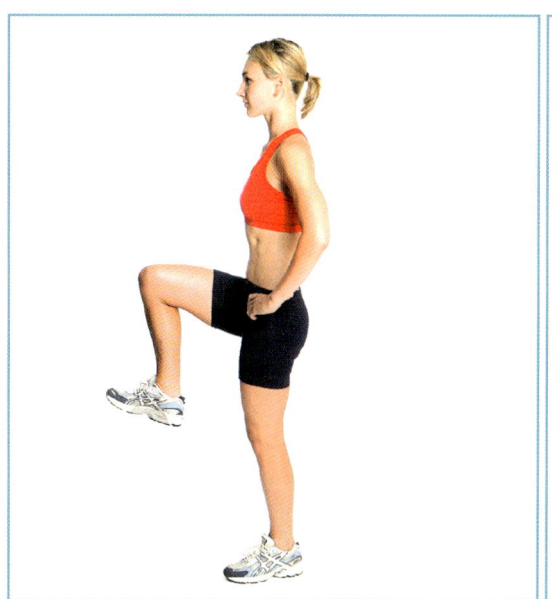

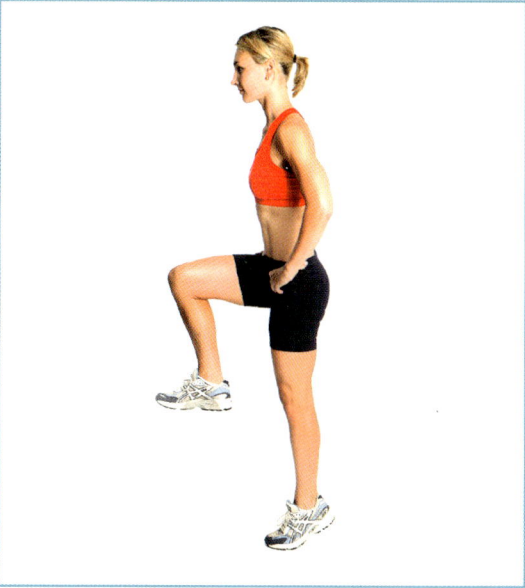

Position:
Stand tall with hands on hips and one knee raised in front of the body. Brace stomach muscles.

Action:
Maintaining good balance, raise up onto toes, then lower. Use chair for balance in initial stages. Repeat with opposite leg.

WAISTLINE WORKOUT

5. Stomach Crunch (Abdominals)

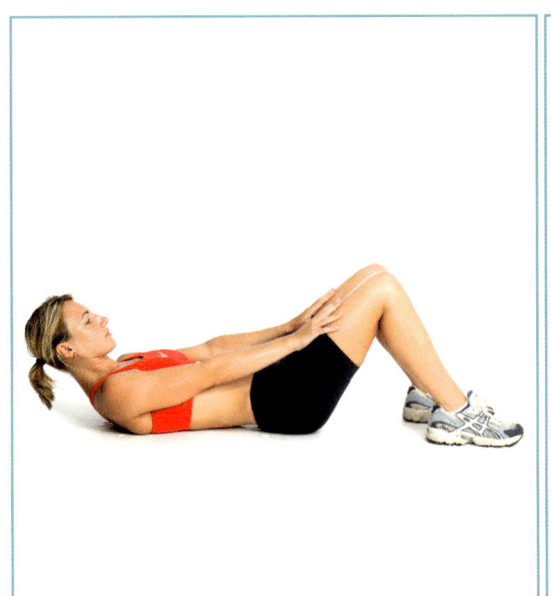

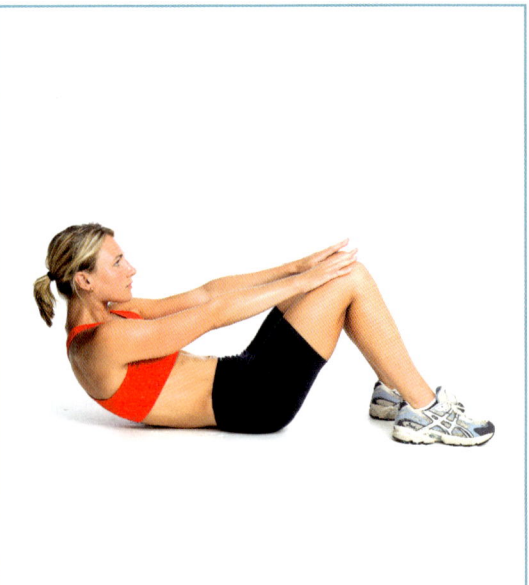

Position:
Lie on back with knees bent and arms extended forward and resting on thighs.

Action:
Raise shoulders off the ground and slide hands up to knees, then lower.

Note: Use a half rolled towel or Lumbatube™ under the lower back to help perform exercise.

6. Cross-Overs (Abdominal Obliques)

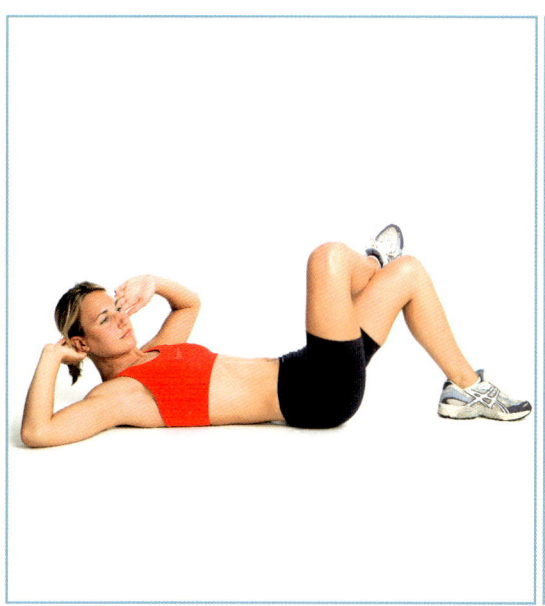

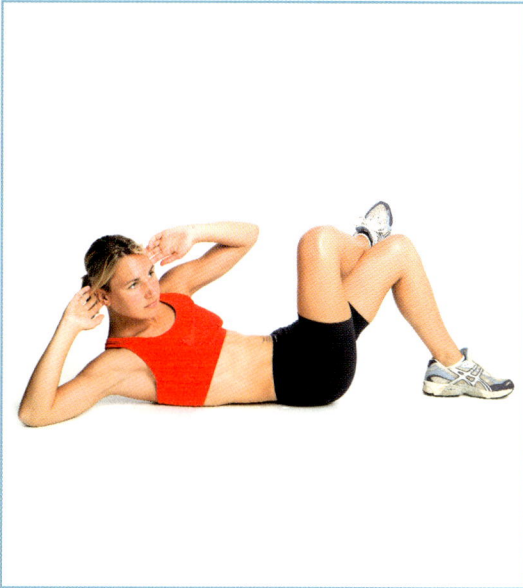

Position:
Lie on back with knees bent and hands resting behind head. Raise right leg and place foot across opposite thigh.

Action:
Raise shoulders and cross left elbow towards right knee, then lower. (Complete set and repeat on opposite side in opposite direction).

Muscle Toning Strength Training - Routine 2

Strength training using weights or machines is important for weight loss, raising your metabolism, burning fat, building muscle and keeping your bones and connective tissue strong. It's a good idea to start with machines and utilize the knowledge of a certified fitness professional or strength and conditioning coach if you exercise at a gym. Machines are generally easier to use and you'll condition your muscles before moving on to free weights, which requires a bit more coordination and the use of more muscles to stabilize your body.

Getting started
- Warm up with 5-10 minutes of light cardiovascular exercise.
- Perform gentle stretches for the whole body.
- Choose one exercise for each muscle group and do 1 set of 10-15 repetitions of each exercise before progressing to 2 or 3 sets over the ensuing weeks.
- Rest 60 seconds between each set.
- Drink at least 2 glasses of water during your workout.
- Start with a program that works all muscle groups and perform 2 or 3 times a week.
- Give yourself at least 24-48 hours to recover before repeating the same exercise.
- The first few weeks, focus on learning how to do each exercise rather than on how much weight you're lifting.
- After 4 or more weeks of consistent strength training, you can change your routine to make it more demanding and/or increase the weight being lifted.
- Stretch between sets and after your workout.
- Cool down with light cardiovascular exercise and gentle stretching routine.
- Apply strength training cycle to progress development (see graph on the next page).

General WW Strength Training Cycles

In the cycle of WW you may apply a 4-week training cycle that changes every 4 weeks as shown in the chart below:

	1. Beginner or restarting	2. General Conditioning	3. Strength
Sets	1-3	1-3	2-5
Reps	12-15	10-12	6-8
Percentage (%) related to a maximum lift	40-50%	50-60%	60-80%
Intensity	low	moderate	high
Volume	moderate	moderate/high	moderate
12-week Training Cycle	Weeks 1-4	Week 5-8	Weeks 9-12

To ensure safe progress with strength training, adhere to the following training guidelines:

- Gain approval to exercise from your doctor, especially if you are pregnant or have a previous injury.
- See a physical therapist to assess your posture and joint mechanics and approve appropriate exercises for you.
- Have a physical therapist or certified trainer demonstrate and supervise each exercise and correct any faults you may have whilst performing them yourself.
- Emphasize quality of movement over quantity.
- Get to know your muscles to understand their function.
- Warm-up the body prior to exercising followed by pre-activity stretching.
- Apply the 3B's Principle™ for helping maintaining correct body posture and maximize your training outcomes.
- Ensure the head and neck maintain a neutral position in line with the lower back at all times.
- If at any stage during exercising you feel tension, numbness, dizziness or pain, stop the exercise immediately and seek medical advice.

Strength Training

Beginner Split Workout

STEP 2

Beginner Split Workout

- Perform exercises in order
- See optional (2nd) exercise for training variety
- Apply 3 strength training cycles (on previous pages) to the vary repetitions, sets, intensity and weight
- Rest 60 seconds in between each exercise

Session 1: Upper Body – 2-3 x week

1. Bench Press
(or Dumbbell Press exercise)

Sets: 2-3
Reps: 10-15
Rest: 60 seconds

Page 94 and 95

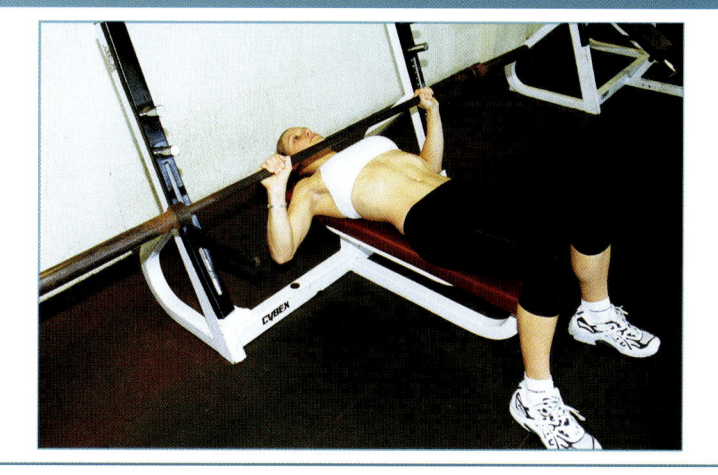

2. Seated Row
(or Lat Pull Down exercise)

Sets: 2-3
Reps: 10-15
Rest: 60 seconds

Page 96 and 97

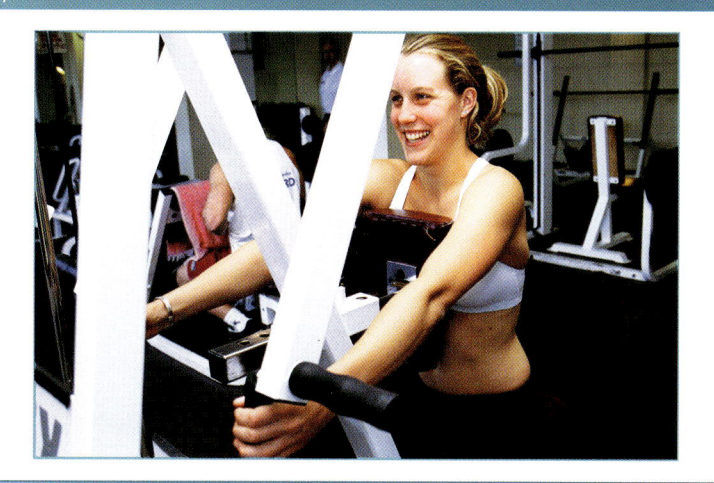

WAISTLINE WORKOUT

3. Dumbbell Biceps Curl
(or Barbell Biceps Curl exercise)

Sets: 2-3
Reps: 10-15
Rest: 60 seconds

Page 98 and 99

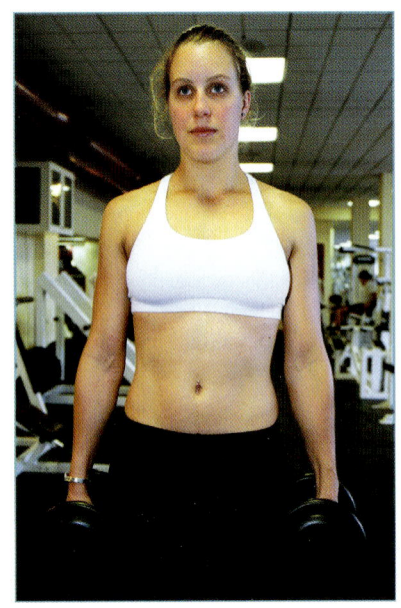

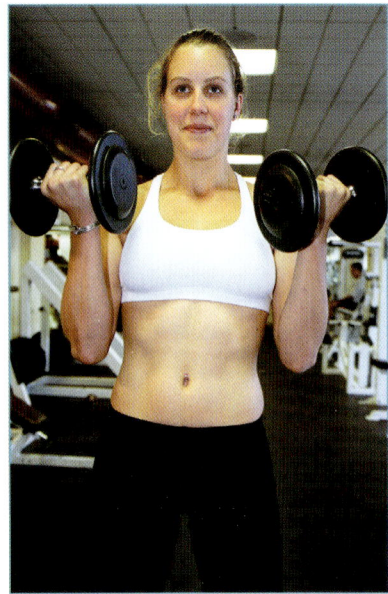

4. Dumbbell Shoulder Press
(or Dumbbell Side Raises)

Sets: 2-3
Reps: 10-15
Rest: 60 seconds

Page 100 and 101

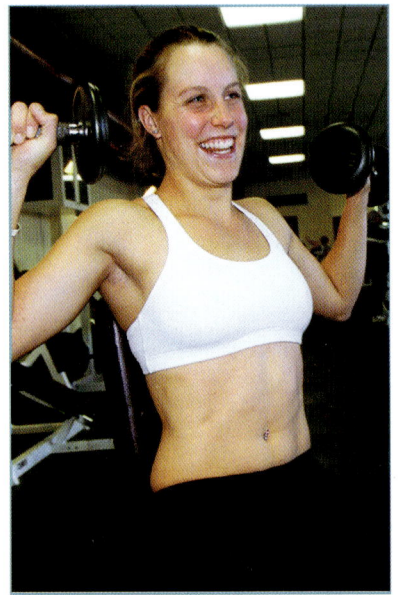

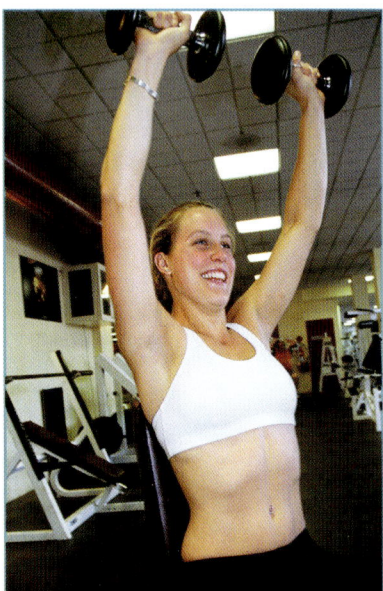

STEP 2

Session 2 – Lower Body and Abdominals – 1-2 x week

1. Leg Press
(or Barbell Squat exercise)

Sets: 2-3
Reps: 10-15
Rest: 60 seconds

Page 102 or 104

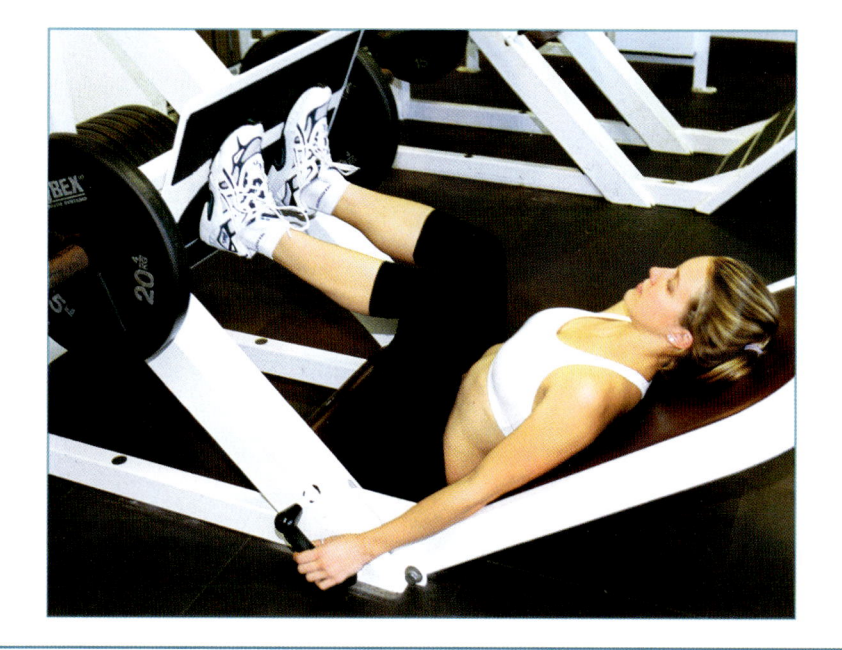

2. Leg Curl

Sets: 2-3
Reps: 10-15
Rest: 60 seconds

Page 105

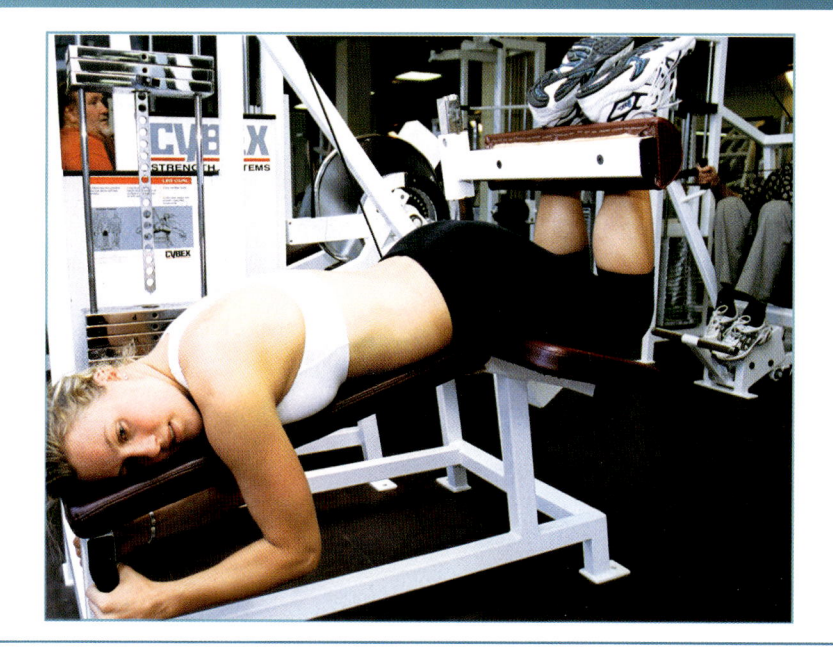

WAISTLINE WORKOUT

3. Leg Extension

Sets: 2-3
Reps: 10-15
Rest: 60 seconds

Page 106

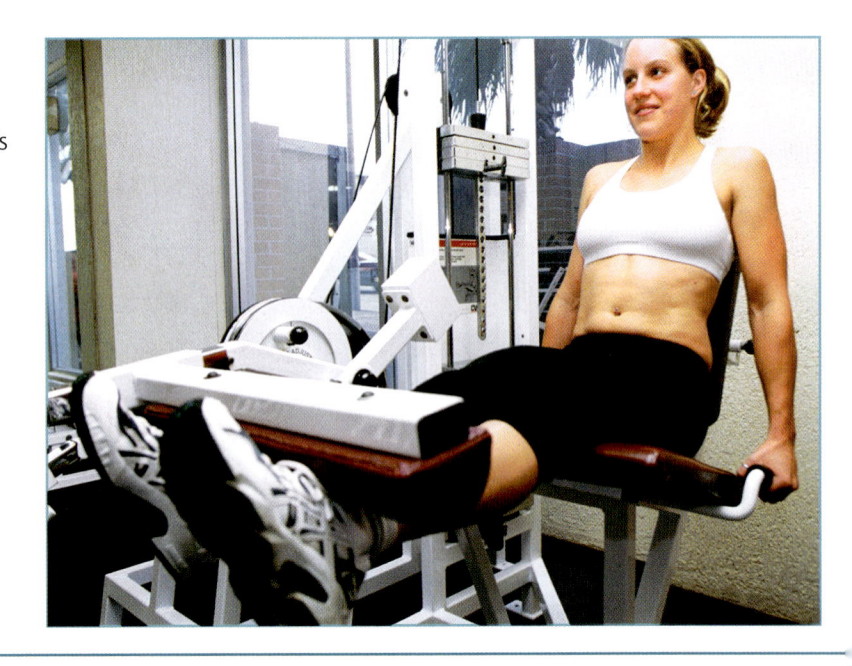

4. Stationary Barbell Lunges
(or Barbell Squat exercise)

Sets: 2 (each leg)
Reps: 10-15
Rest: 60 seconds

Page 103 or 104

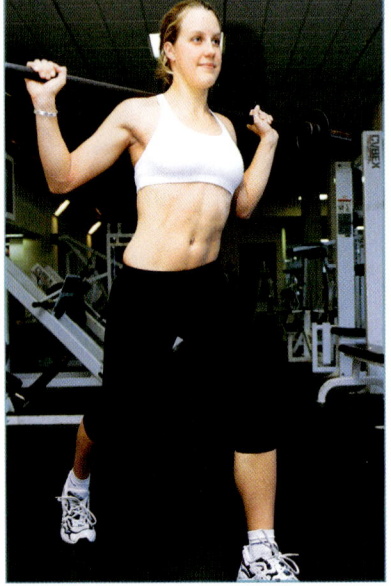

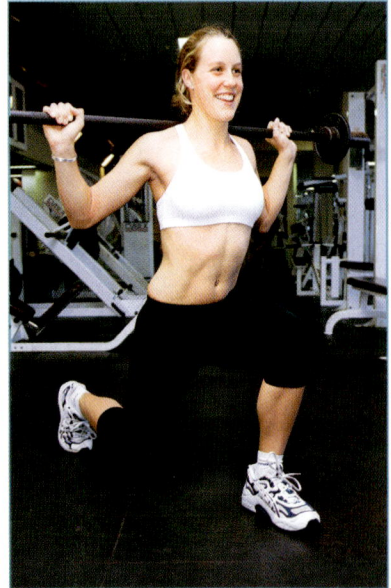

STEP 2

5. Fitness Ball Abdominal Crunch

Sets: 2-3
Reps: 10-15
Rest: 60 seconds

Page 107

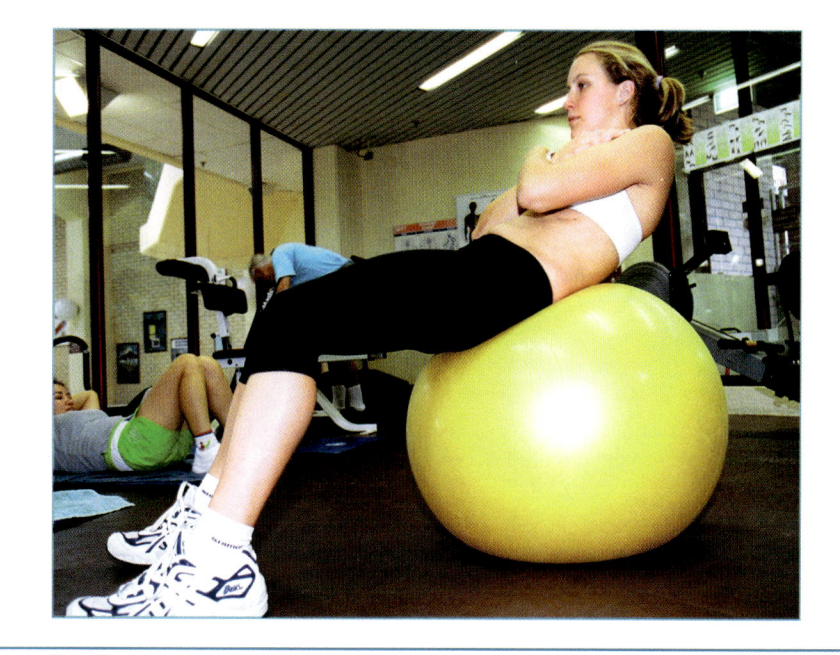

6. Elbow to Knee

Sets: 2-3 (each side)
Reps: 10-15
Rest: Nil;
move directly from one side to the other

Page 83

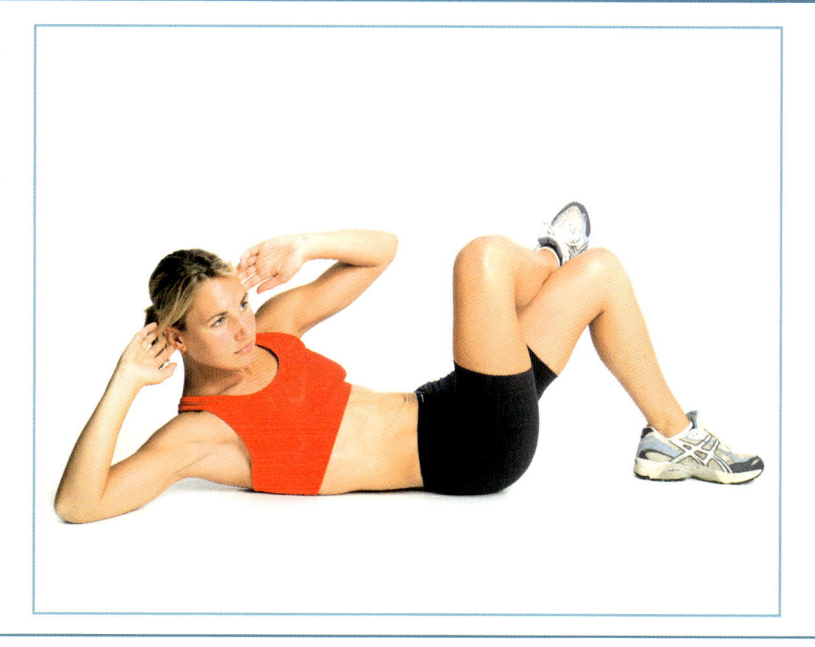

7. Lower Leg Raises

Sets: 2-3
Reps: 10-15
Rest: 60 seconds

Page 108

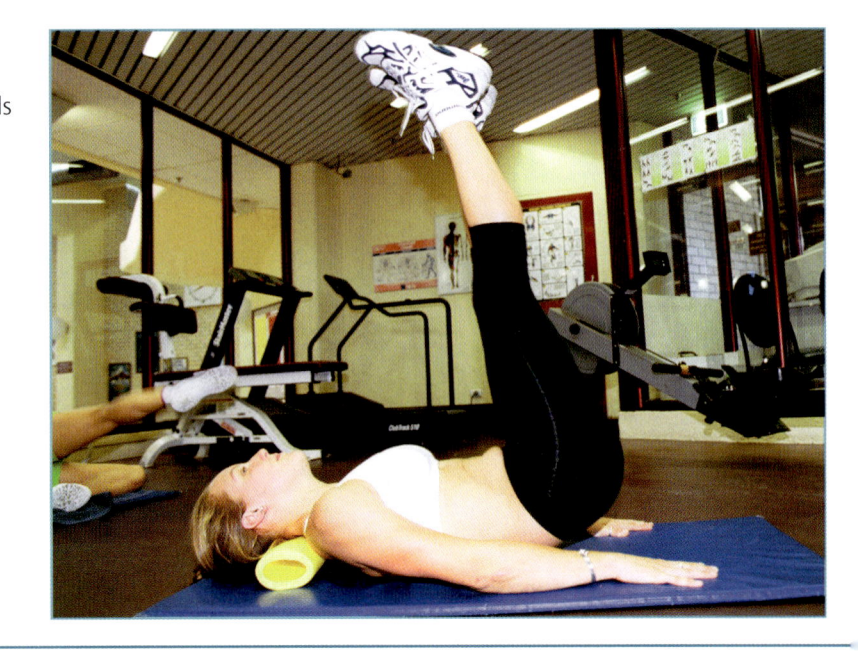

Strength Training

Exercise Descriptions

WAISTLINE WORKOUT

Exercise: Bench Press

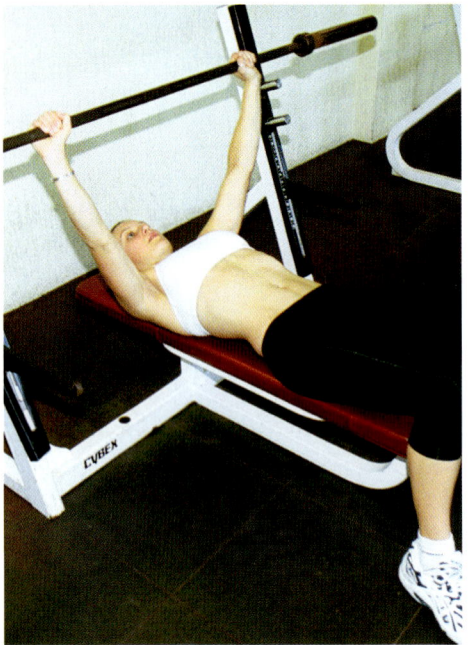

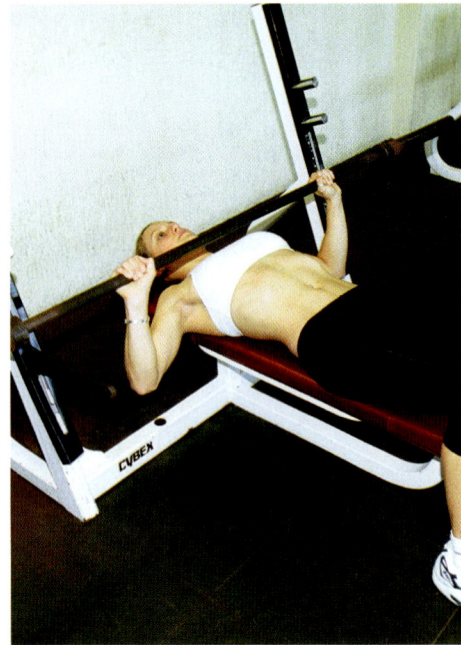

Start Position   Midpoint

Description
- Lie on your back on flat bench.
- Grip bar evenly about shoulder-width apart.
- Maintaining the natural curve of your lower back, brace your stomach.
- Apply 3B's Principle™ - Brace, Breath and Body Position.
- Breathe in as you lower the barbell to the midline of your chest.
- Breathe out as you press the barbell to arm's length.
- Maintain a continuous flowing movement at all times until repetitions completed.

STEP 2

Exercise: Dumbbell Press

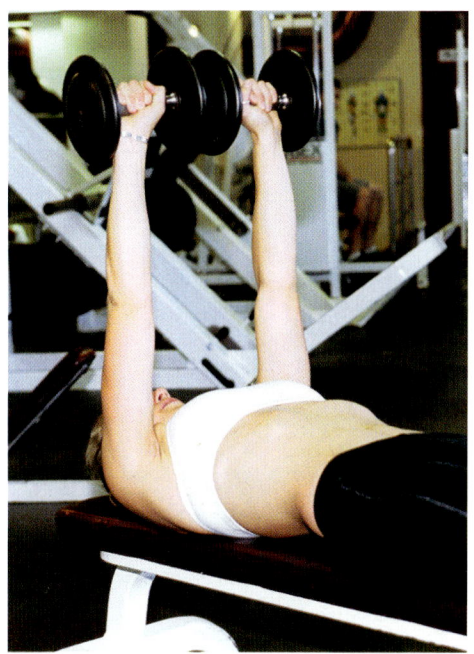

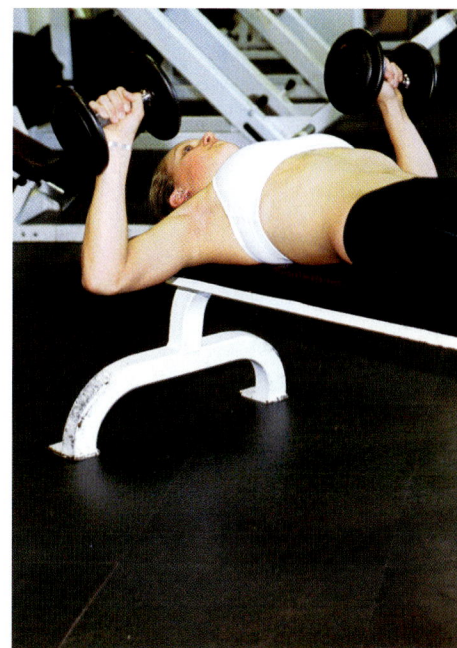

Start Position   Midpoint

Description
- Lie on your back on a flat bench.
- Grip dumbbells evenly and raise into air together above chest midline, palms facing towards knees.
- Maintaining the natural curve of your lower back, brace your stomach.
- Apply 3B's Principle™ - Brace, Breath and Body Position.
- Breathe in as you simultaneously separate and lower the dumbbells in an arch motion to the side of the body, keeping in line with your chest.
- Breathe out as you press the dumbbells to arm's length back together.
- Maintain a continuous flowing movement at all times until repetitions completed.

WAISTLINE WORKOUT

Exercise: Seated Row

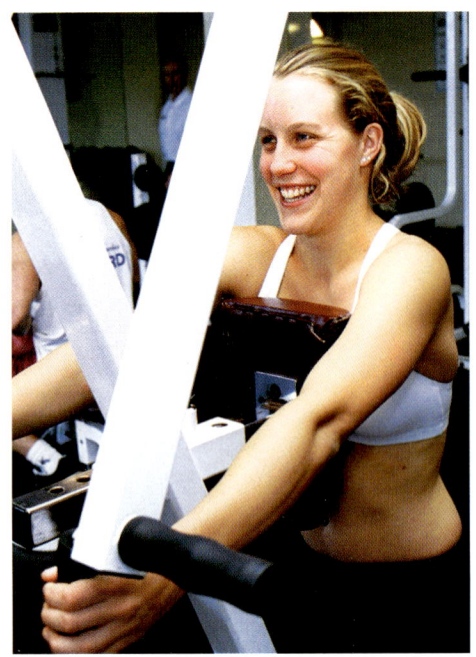

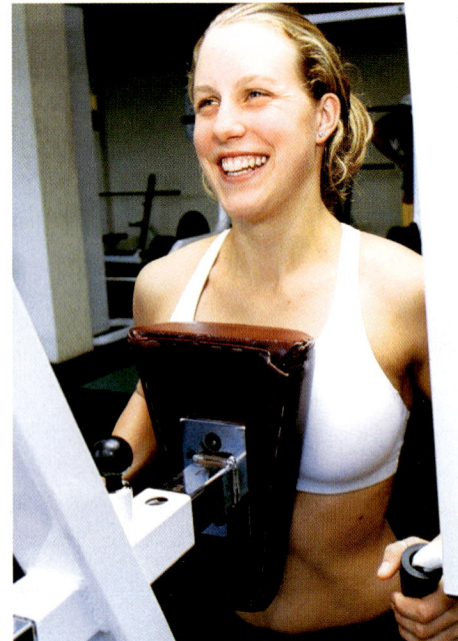

Start Position | Midpoint

Description
- Sit forwards on seated row machine and then adjust height of seat and chest pad to fit appropriately.
- With arms at full length hold onto handles.
- Apply 3B's Principle™ - Brace, Breath and Body Position.
- Breathe out as you bend your elbows and pull the handles back by your side.
- Breathe in and return arms towards starting position.
- Maintain a continuous flowing movement at all times up repetitions completed.

STEP 2

Exercise: Lat Pull Down

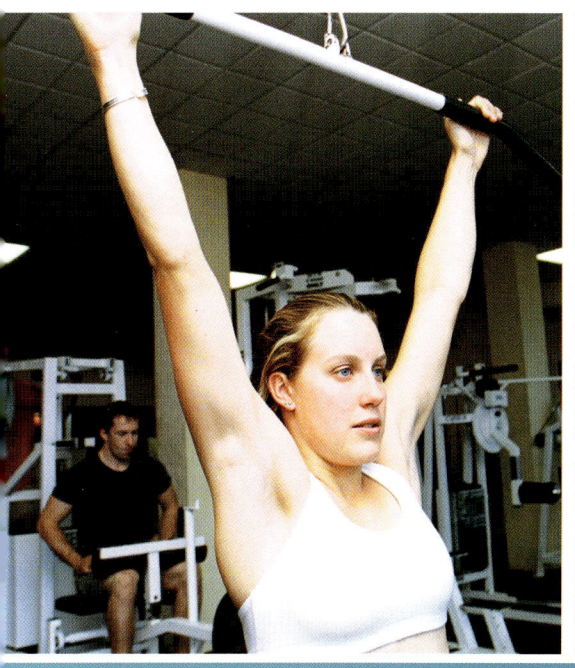

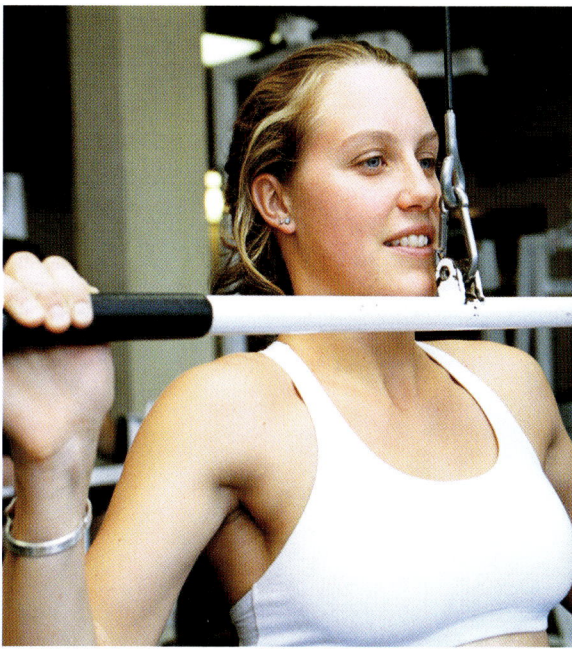

Start Position   Midpoint

Description
- Take an overhand grip on bar overhead, wrists straight.
- Sit with your back straight, chest lifted and head in line with your spine.
- Maintaining the natural curve of your lower back, brace your stomach.
- Apply 3B's Principle™ - Brace, Breath and Body Position.
- Breathe out as you pull the bar down towards your chest by leaning slightly backwards.
- Breathe in as you allow the bar to return to upright position in a controlled manner.
- Keep the overhead bar moving at all times in an even and controlled manner in time with your deep breathing.

WAISTLINE WORKOUT

Exercise: Dumbbell Biceps Curl

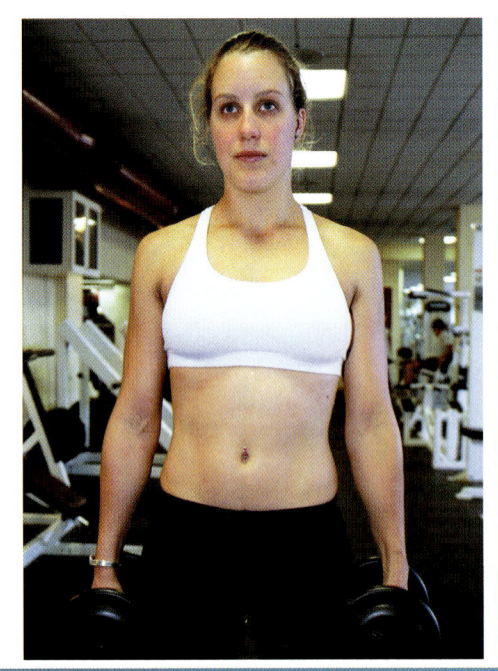

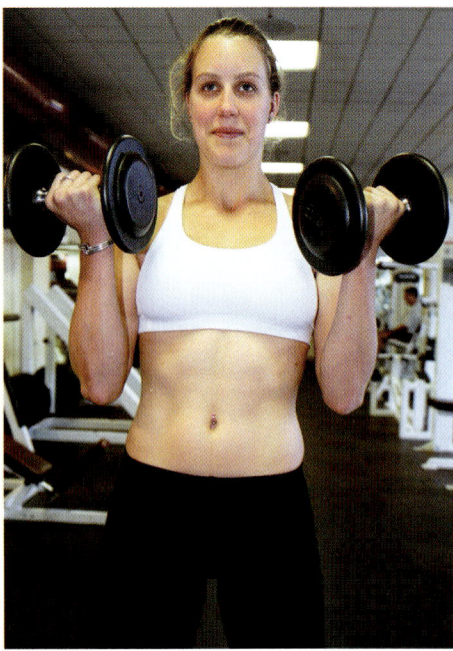

Start Position   Midpoint

Description
- Stand with your back straight and feet shoulder width apart, knees slightly bent.
- Hold dumbbells at arm's length by your side. Tuck your upper arms into your body, whilst keeping your wrists straight.
- Maintaining the natural curve of your lower back, brace your stomach.
- Apply 3B's Principle™ - Brace, Breath and Body Position.
- Breathe out as you bend your elbows and draw the dumbbells simultaneously to shoulder height, twisting the dumbbell as you raise your arm with palms facing towards body.
- Breathe in as you lower the dumbbells to the side of your body.
- Maintain a continuous flowing movement at all times until repetitions completed.
- **Variation:** Alternate one arm up and down, then the other for a single arm curl.

STEP 2

Exercise: Barbell Biceps Curl

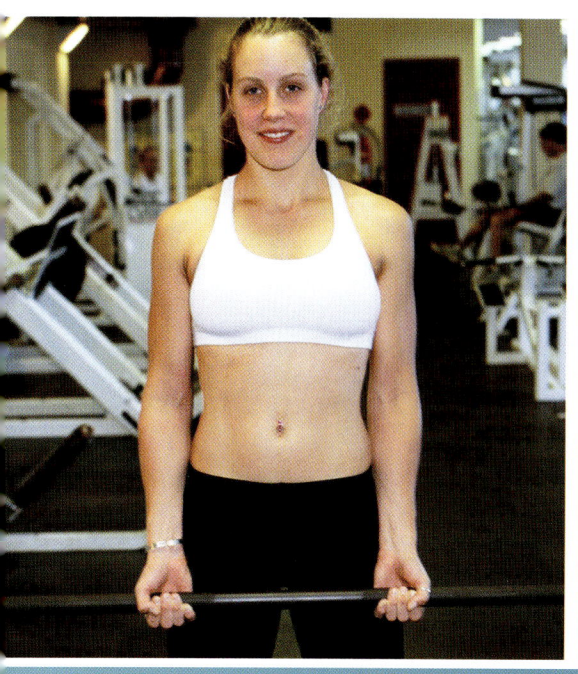

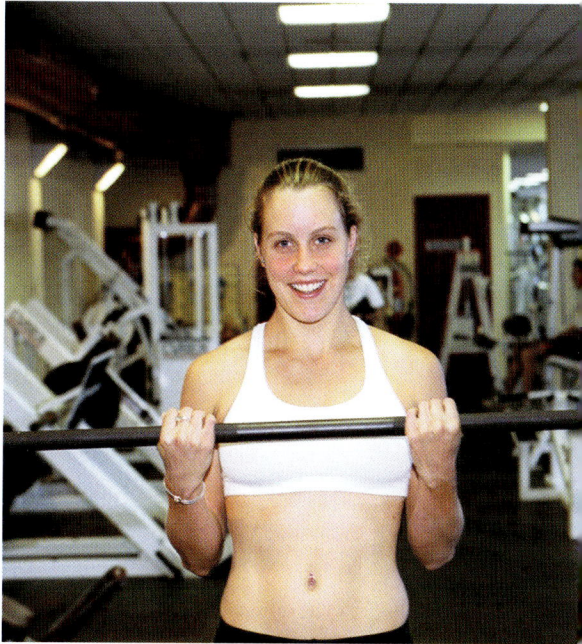

Start Position   Midpoint

Description
- Stand with your back straight and feet shoulder width apart, knees slightly bent.
- With your hands shoulder width apart, take an underhand grip on barbell and rest on the front of your thighs.
- Tuck your upper arms into your body, whilst keeping your wrists straight.
- Maintaining the natural curve of your lower back, brace your stomach.
- Apply 3B's Principle™ - Brace, Breath and Body Position.
- Breathe out as you bend your elbows and draw the bar to shoulder height – keeping your elbows close to the body.
- Breathe in as you lower the bars to your thighs.
- Maintain a continuous flowing movement at all times until repetitions completed.

WAISTLINE WORKOUT

Exercise: Dumbbell Shoulder Press

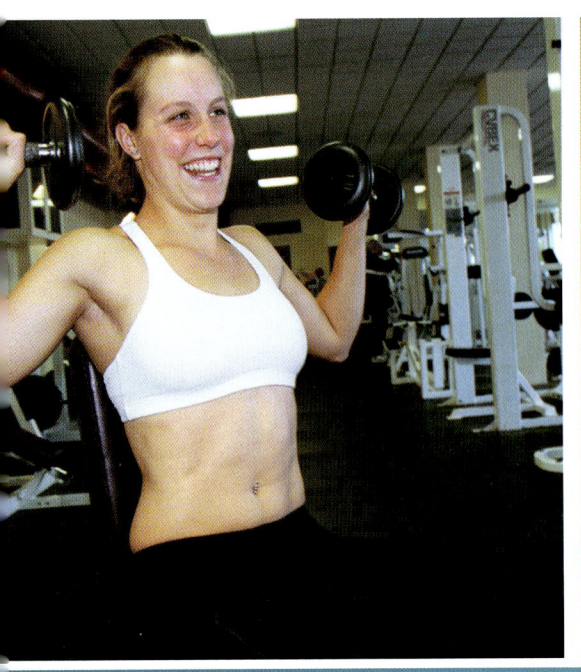

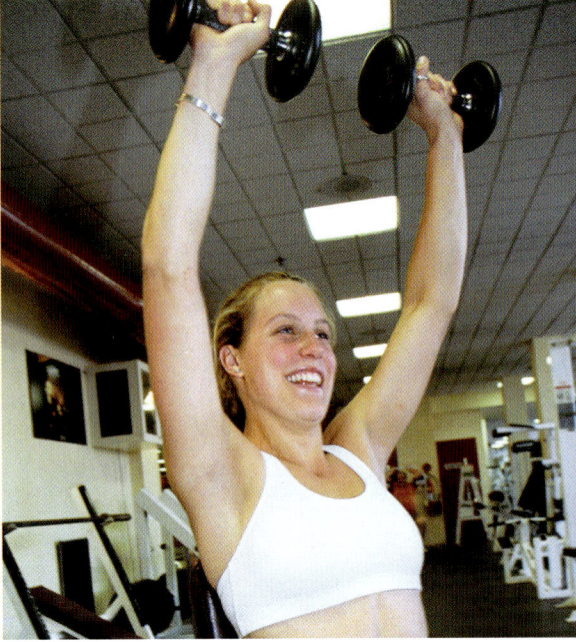

Start Position   Midpoint

Description
- Sit with your back straight, head in line with your spine and feet shoulder width apart.
- Grip dumbbells and lift to shoulder height, palms facing forward and wrists straight.
- Maintaining the natural curve of your lower back, brace your stomach.
- Apply 3B's Principle™ - Brace, Breath and Body Position.
- Breathe out as you press the dumbbells to arm's length overhead and together.
- Breathe in as you lower the dumbbells to shoulder height.
- Maintain a continuous flowing movement at all times until repetitions completed.
- Resist any arching of the lower back, by keeping stomach braced.

STEP 2

Exercise: Dumbbell Side Raises

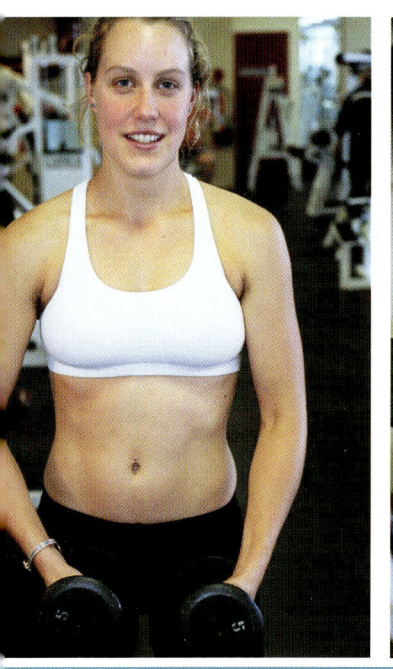

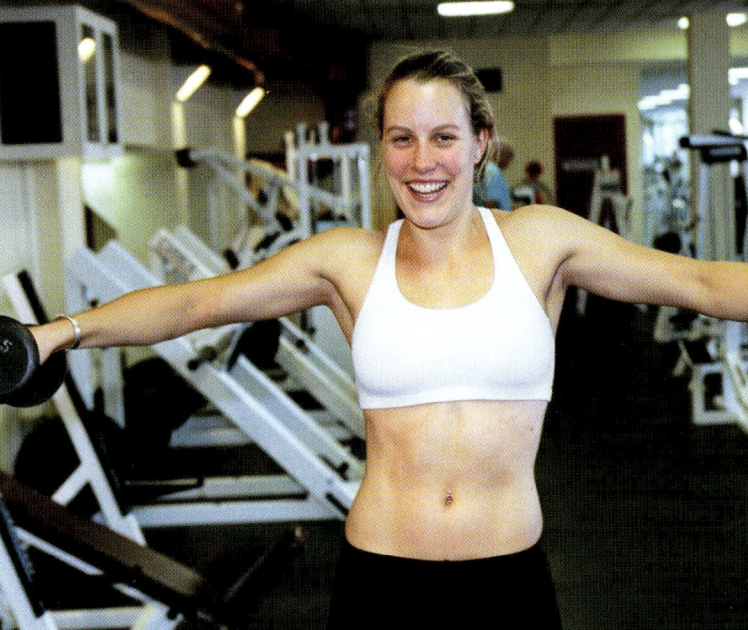

Start Position   Midpoint

Description
- Stand with your back straight and feet shoulder width apart, knees slightly bent.
- Grip dumbbells and raise to the front of your thighs, arms slightly bent, palms facing together, wrists straight.
- Maintaining the natural curve of your lower back, brace your stomach.
- Apply 3B's Principle™ - Brace, Breath and Body Position.
- Breathe out as you extend your arms simultaneously out to the side in a semi-circle, leading with your elbows and knuckles to shoulder level.
- Breathe in as you lower the dumbbells to the front of your body in a controlled manner.
- Maintain a continuous flowing movement at all times until repetitions completed.
- **Note:** Bend arms slightly to reduce stress and load when beginning.

WAISTLINE WORKOUT

Exercise: Leg Press

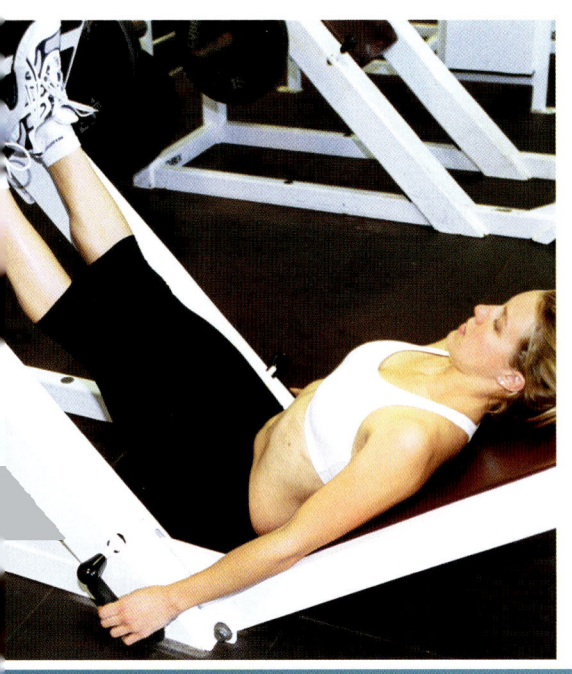

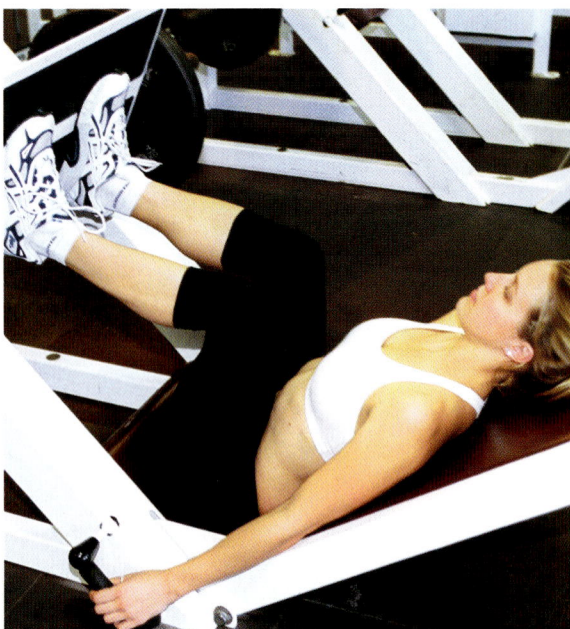

Start Position | Midpoint

Description
- Sit in leg press machine and place feet shoulder-width apart on platform.
- Maintaining the natural curve of your lower back, brace your stomach.
- Apply 3B's Principle™ - Brace, Breath and Body Position.
- Extend legs and release safety attachment of machine with hands to allow free movement
- Breathe in, lowering your legs at your knees.
- Breathe out as you press and extend the legs away from the body.
- Maintain a continuous flowing movement at all times until repetitions completed.

Exercise: Stationary Barbell Lunges

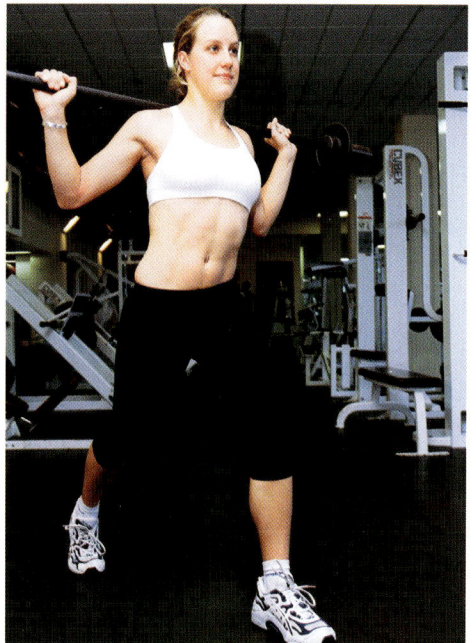

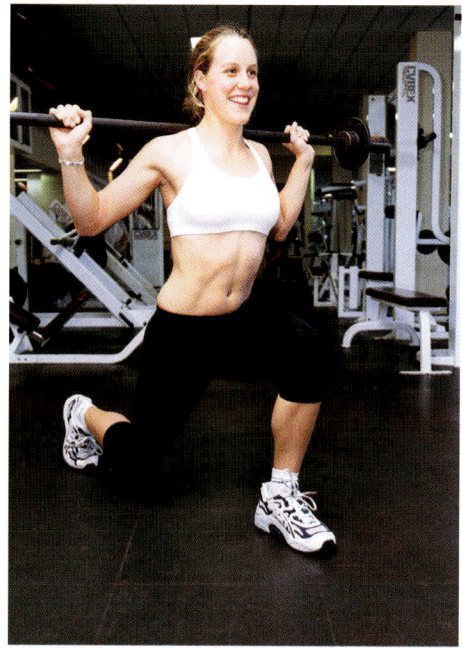

Start Position | Midpoint

Description
- Stand in forward lunge position, one foot forward and the other back with legs slightly bent – barbell resting across shoulders.
- Maintaining the natural curve of your lower back, brace your stomach.
- Apply 3B's Principle™ – Brace, Breath and Body Position.
- Breathe in as lower your rear knee towards the ground.
- Breathe out as you rise up.
- Maintain a continuous flowing movement at all times until repetitions completed.
- Repeat action with opposite leg.
- **Variety:** (1) Use hand weights held down by side; (2) Alternate leg lunges forwards and back.

WAISTLINE WORKOUT

Exercise: Barbell Squat

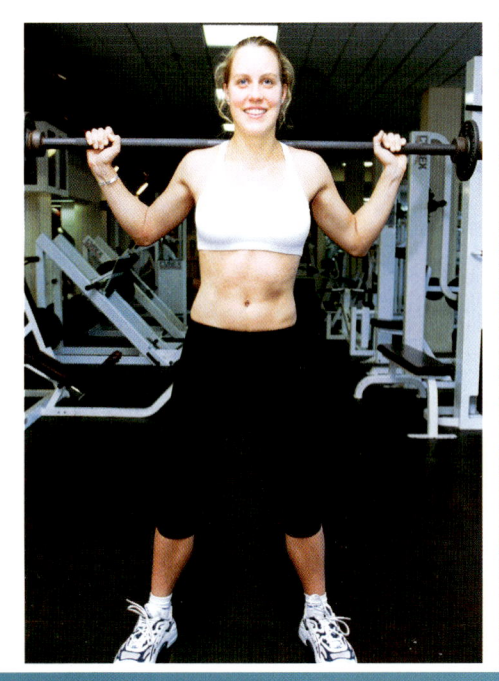

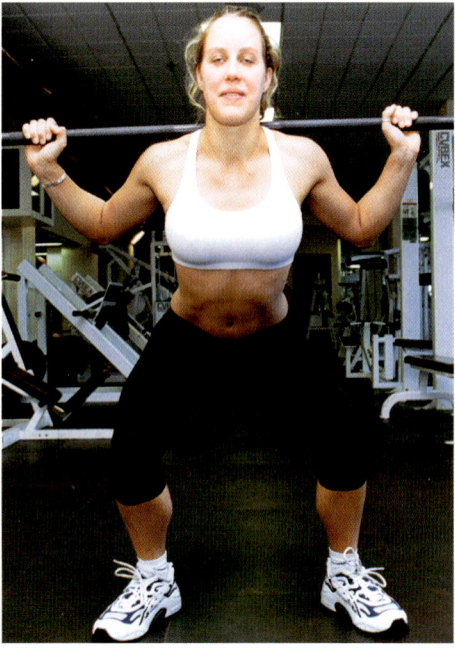

Start Position | Midpoint

Description
- Stand with feet shoulder width apart and bar resting across rear of shoulders.
- Maintaining the natural curve of your lower back, brace your stomach.
- Apply 3B's Principle™ - Brace, Breath and Body Position
- Breathe in as you slowly bend at your knees, sit back and lower buttocks towards the ground until legs are at a 90-degree angle.
- Breathe out as you raise your body upwards using your legs to starting position.
- Maintain a continuous flowing movement at all times until repetitions completed.
- **Note:** Keep your heels on the floor and resist leaning forward from the hips. Maintain ear over shoulder, over hip over ankle – from side position – and knees following the line of the toes.

Exercise: Leg Curl

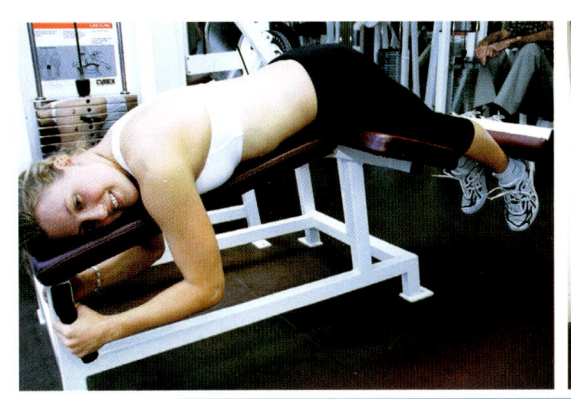

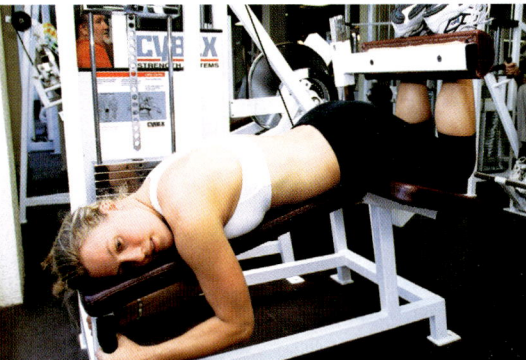

Start Position   Midpoint

Description
- Lie face down with lower calf and heel region placed under roller pad.
- Maintaining the natural curve of your lower back, brace your stomach.
- Apply 3B's Principle™ - Brace, Breath and Body Position.
- Breathe out as you bend your knees and curl your feet toward your buttocks – keeping your hips firmly on the bench.
- Breathe in as you lower your legs towards starting position.
- Avoid the weighted stack touching or body relaxing.
- Maintain a continuous flowing movement at all times until repetitions completed.

WAISTLINE WORKOUT

Exercise: Leg Extension

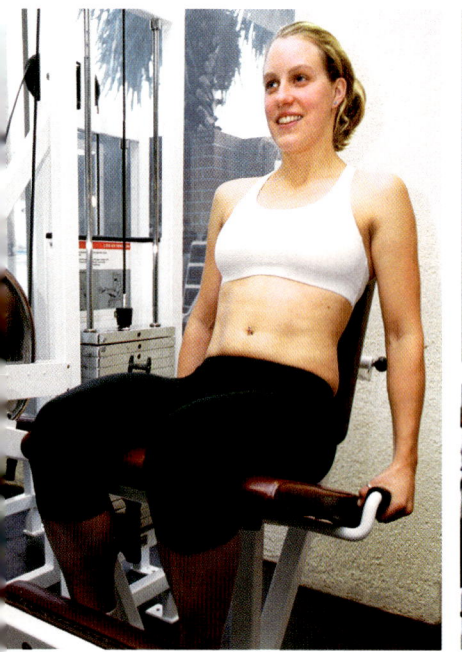

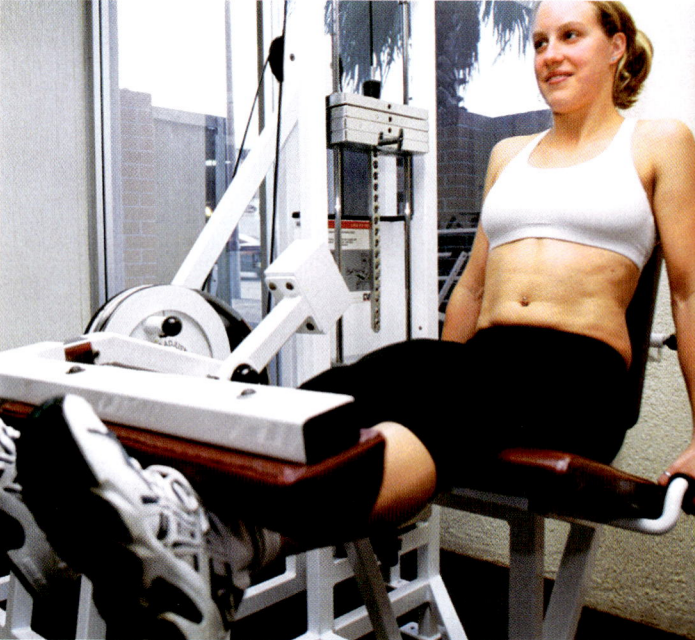

Start Position | Midpoint

Description
- Sit in machine with shin region resting against pads – adjust appropriately – and flex feet by pulling toes up towards shin and hold.
- Adjust back rest so bent leg (back of knee) is resting on edge of seat.
- Maintaining the natural curve of your lower back, brace your stomach.
- Apply 3B's Principle™ - Brace, Breath and Body Position.
- Breathe out as you extend the legs forward until straight.
- Breathe in as you lower your legs leading with your heels.
- Avoid the weighted stack touching or body relaxing.
- Maintain a continuous flowing movement at all times until repetitions completed.

STEP 2

Exercise: Fitness Ball Crunch

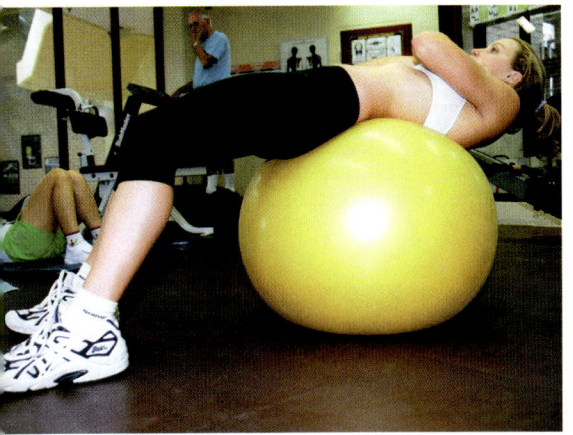

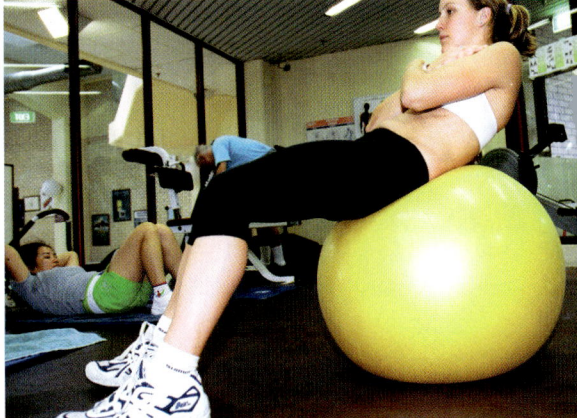

Start Position   **Midpoint**

Description
- Lie on your back on Fitness Ball with your feet shoulder width apart, knees bent at 90 degrees and arms resting across chest.
- Apply 3B's Principle™ - Brace, Breath and Body Position.
- Breathe out as you lift your shoulders, crunching your chest towards your hips.
- Breathe in as you lower your shoulders back down onto to the ball.
- Avoid relaxing stomach muscles. Keep the tension on the stomach at all times until all repetitions are complete.
- **Note:** Rest arms behind head or extend to increase exercise intensity.

WAISTLINE WORKOUT

Exercise: Lower Leg Raises

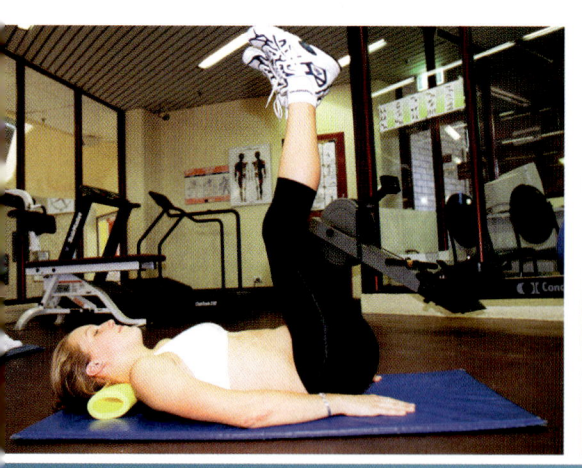

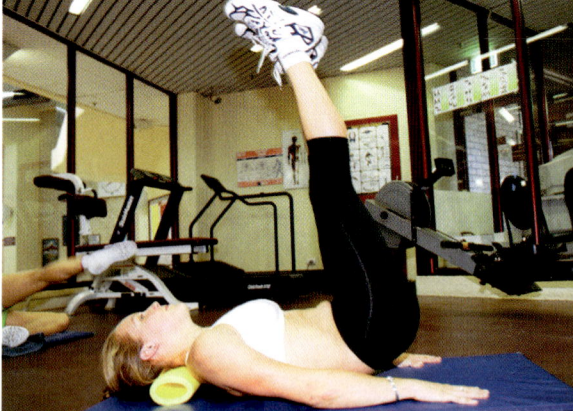

Start Position | **Midpoint**

Description
- Lie on your back with your legs vertical in the air and slightly bent with hands beside (or under) your buttocks and rolled towel or LumbAtube™ placed under your neck for support.
- Apply 3B's Principle™ - Brace, Breath and Body Position.
- Breathe out as you activate your abdominal muscles (pulling inwards), lifting your lower back and hips off the ground with feet raising towards the ceiling – resist swinging the legs forwards or backwards.
- Breathe in as you lower towards the ground, keeping the tension on the stomach at all times until repetitions are completed.

© fotolia, EastWest Imaging

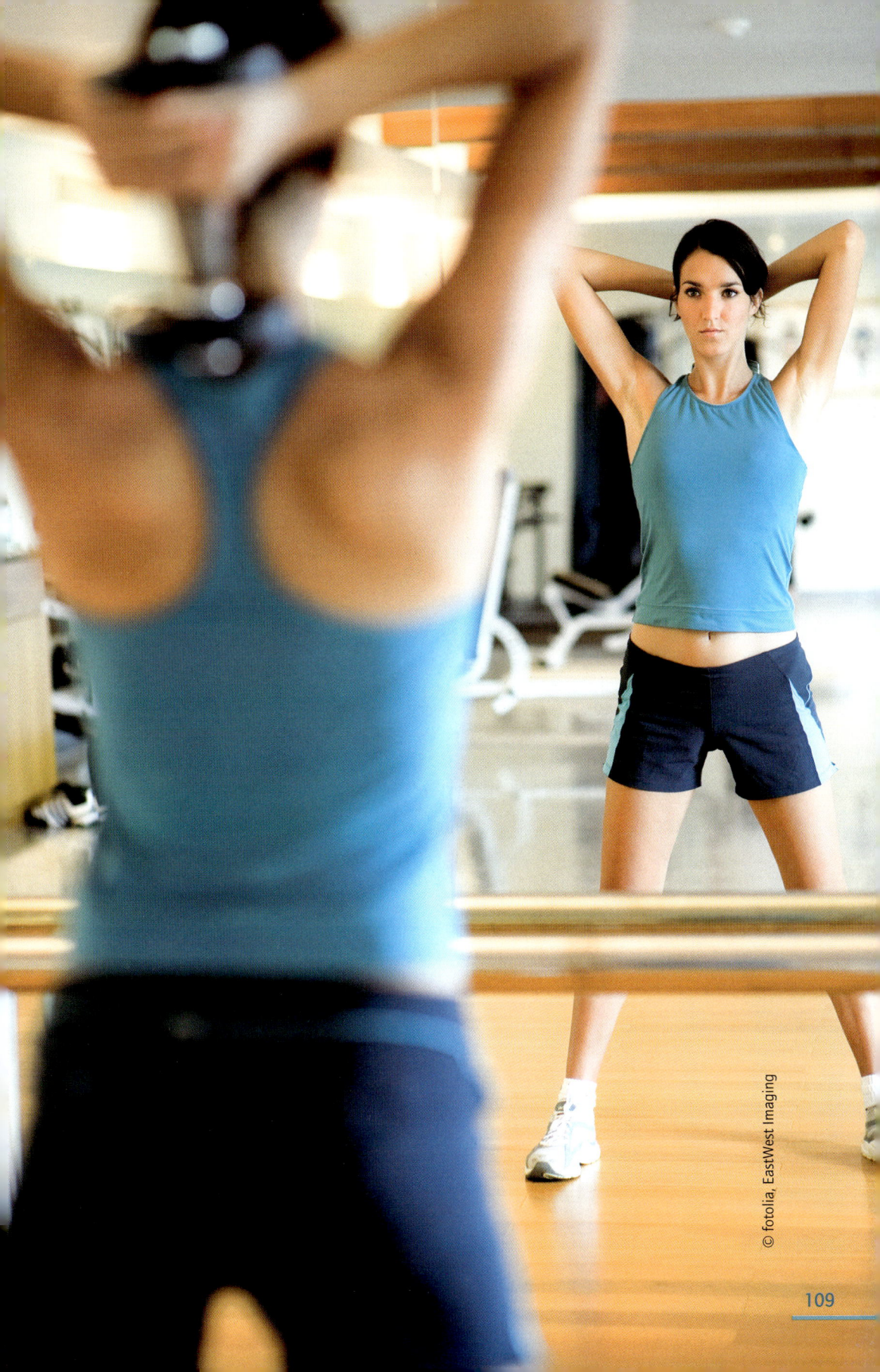

109

Phase 2: Heart & Lung (Cardiovascular) Fitness

Increasing your level of daily movement will not only help reduce the amount of fat your body is carrying, it will also improve the function of your heart and lungs and your fitness levels. Cardiovascular (aerobic) activity is defined as 'prolonged continuous movement of large muscle groups' that increases one's heart rate. That means something that keeps you moving, constantly, such as brisk walking or cycling for an extended period of time such as 20-60 minutes. It may be appropriate for some people to start with a shorter exercise period, when first starting out; be guided by your doctor. When you exercise, your effort must exceed that of your normal daily activities. As the exercises become easier, the intensity needs to be gradually increased. A few other examples of cardiovascular exercise include brisk walking, jogging, cycling, boxing, rowing, swimming and dancing.

Wherever you stand today in terms of your health, it's a good idea to be more active instead of sitting around. If there's not much movement in your day, you can be quite sure that there will be more energy going into your body from food than is going out. To correct this energy imbalance, all movement counts in terms of burning calories. So, being more active or moving quicker in and around the house and with your daily activities can all help towards stripping that extra fat from your abdominal and thigh region.

Starting Point

When first starting out, walking is the answer, because it's one of the safest exercises you can do for your body. A regular walking routine can do a world of preventative good, from lowering your risk of diabetes, stroke and osteoporosis to reducing high blood pressure, treating arthritis and even depression. Most importantly, brisk walking is good for your heart as it keeps it in shape for pumping blood around the body and increasing oxygen consumption.
If you haven't exercised in a while, the aim is to introduce a realistic approach that involves progression of time, volume and intensity. Walking works when starting back because the first thing you'll notice if its been a while since you last exercised is a how quickly and how high your heart starts racing. Walking helps to keep this under control. There's less stress of your joints and you can rest at any time. As you continue with your exercise program, your fitness level will improve and your resting pulse should be lowered. But before you get started, visit your doctor to discuss which exercise and exercise intensity is right for you as well as gaining medical clearance to get under way.

Understanding Your Heart Rate

Becoming familiar with how your body responds to exercise is important in the initial phases. Understanding how your heart rate responds to movement and exercise allows you to monitor how hard you are working. When you're unfit, the heart will be weaker and has to work harder to circulate blood to the muscles than someone who is fit. Women starting out for the first time or returning to exercise after a long break should start at a relatively comfortable level and gradually increase the duration and intensity as you become fitter and your heart adapts.

Getting to know your heart rate (or pulse) is a good measure of how hard you are working. Your resting pulse refers to how fast your heart rate is beating per minute at rest. For most people it is around 60-72 beats per minute. For those who are fitter it can be lower. At the other end of the scale there is a maximum heart rate (MHR) that is calculated in general terms by deducting 220 minus your age (in years). For example, if you are 45 it would be calculated as: 220 − 45 = 175 beats per minute. For general fitness, you need to work at a range between 60–75% of your maximum heart rate (MHR). Above this level is relative to those in competitive sport or extremely fit individuals. The more weight you carry, the harder your heart will have to work initially, so take it easy for the first few weeks gradually adding a few minutes to your routine at a time.

The following chart outlines the heart rate exercise range relative to your age:

Age	60% of MHR range in beats per minute	75% of MHR range in beats per minute	Maximum Heart Rate (MHR) in beats per minute
20	120	150	200
25	117	146	195
30	114	142	190
35	111	138	185
40	108	135	180
45	105	131	175
50	102	128	170
55	99	124	165
60	96	120	160
65	93	116	155

You can take your resting pulse before you start to exercise as well as during and after your workout to see what pulse rate per minute you are working at and whether to speed up or slow down. To do this, place your first two fingers either on your upturned wrist or your neck and count the beats for 60 seconds. Alternatively, count the beats for 15 seconds and multiply by 4 to calculate your pulse rate per minute. For example, if your pulse rate is 30 beats in 15 seconds, it will be 120 (30 x 4) over a minute. Monitoring your heart way is a great way to progressively develop your fitness level without overdoing it. There are also electronic heart rate monitors available that make gauging your pace much easier.

Cardiovascular Exercise Variety

What seems hard for some may not be hard for others, that's why varying the frequency, intensity, time and type (FITT principle) of exercise makes all the difference. If you're in a

WAISTLINE WORKOUT

position where you can already walk for over one hour and are still holding weight around the abdominals and thighs, there's five things you can do:

1. Add strength training into your routine.
2. Varying the intensity (speed and gradient of terrain) when you walk and actually reduce the overall time.
3. Introduce another cardiovascular exercise into your routine that challenges you such as cycling, jogging or indoor rowing machine.
4. Improve you dietary intake as part of the RDI plan.
5. Introduce more incidental movement throughout the day.

In some cases it becomes a role reversal where if you perform plenty of cardiovascular exercise, you need to start strength training. Whilst on the other hand, if you strength train regularly you'll have to introduce cardiovascular training. Or combine both – it can be that simple! Some cardiovascular exercises choices for future use may include:

- Brisk walking
- Jogging
- Aqua Aerobics
- Cross-Trainer
- Step Machine
- Resistance Bands

- Bush walking
- Treadmill
- Dancing
- Elliptical Machine
- Aerobics class
- Exercise DVD

- Hill Walking
- Cycling
- Indoor Rowing
- Stationary Bike
- Boxing or Skipping
- Other: _____

For more details, visit www.thebodycoach.com

Becoming a WW Gold Medallist

WW takes a unique approach compared to other weight loss programs for a reason. To refresh your mind, the primary focus is regaining body symmetry through strength training of the upper body region. To help keep the metabolic rate high and muscles toned throughout the rest of the body, it also includes a strength training routine for the mid and lower body along with essential cardiovascular exercise for improving heart and lung fitness – brisk walking the first choice. By thinking of WW as its own sport, knowing that every sport trains differently to accommodate their specific needs, you can begin to understand why we apply this unique approach that has one goal in mind: achieving your best body shape ever, or in sporting terms becoming a WW Gold Medallist.

Before we look that far ahead, there are a few key elements you need to understand. In any sports there are a 4 key periods: pre-season, in-season, finals and post-season recovery. I'd be honest in saying that if you are reading this book; your post season has most likely been an extended one or that you've started a few pre-season training programs but never reached in-season. I see it a lot as a coach and realize for any program to be successful you need to have an objective and a plan and be accountable to it or to someone. For instance, you can't expect not to train, then show up to games on the weekend and expect to play well. Instead, you're more likely to get injured. Regular training and practice on the other hand is what keeps you in shape.

Because you're now about to resume pre-season training, you need to make a commitment to yourself that you're going to stick to the 12-week season, even through hard times. Pre-season is a period where you learn new skills, improve rusty ones, build up your fitness levels and confidence and build new habits. Your pre-season is only 4-weeks, with a further 2 x 4-week cycles for competition and finals. No one ever said it was going to be easy, but one thing is for sure everyone faces similar circumstances and you, yes you, are the only one who can turn this around and make it happen. By providing you with your long term vision, I want you to close your eyes for a few seconds and imagine that gold medal being placed around your neck at the end of the season and how proud and how much healthier you'll be. I want you to use this as your vision throughout your journey to keep you motivated.

Body Coach® 30-Minute WW Cardio Approach

The Body Coach® WW approach to cardio training is a strategic one that involves a 'cycle of intensity' during each session. What this means is that the traditional 1-2 hour long walks many people endure themselves to can now be cut down to as little as 30 minutes, as long as incidental movement is continued throughout the day. This does not mean to say that if you enjoy walking for long periods to stop, quite the contrary. Instead, what I'm about to show you is a way to maximize your valuable time, with extra time for strength training.

Your body is an amazing engine that adapts quickly to the demands placed upon it. In which case, a traditional viewpoint has many people thinking that they have to keep extending the time frame of a training session to reap any benefits. This may be true in a particular way,

WAISTLINE WORKOUT

because more movement is good for your health. The problem is that what started out as a 20 minute walk six-months ago has may have become 90 minutes long and these people are still not achieving the body shape they desire. So, let me share a few secrets with you!

As the body adapts quickly to the demands placed upon it, you need to continually surprise your body in terms of these demands so it has to make changes. In my industry I see a lot of people who train at the same pace day in, day out whether it's swimming laps in the pool, lifting weights or running. In a way, it's like saying they're always idling in one gear. Whilst I praise their efforts and their routine, a few simple changes through the gears with speed variables throughout their training session and all of a sudden immense improvements start to occur. Using different gears and speed variables is the approach we will be using during your 30-minute cardio workout. The most important thing to remember is that some days staying in one gear at one speed and going for shorter or longer periods of time is okay! This is because every little bit of movement counts. The main thing to remember is that when you work with a plan and strategy, everything else in your life seems to benefit also. You become more confident, more organized and more motivated because you know what you are doing and for how long. So, now is the time for change!

Body Coach® WW Power Walking Plan

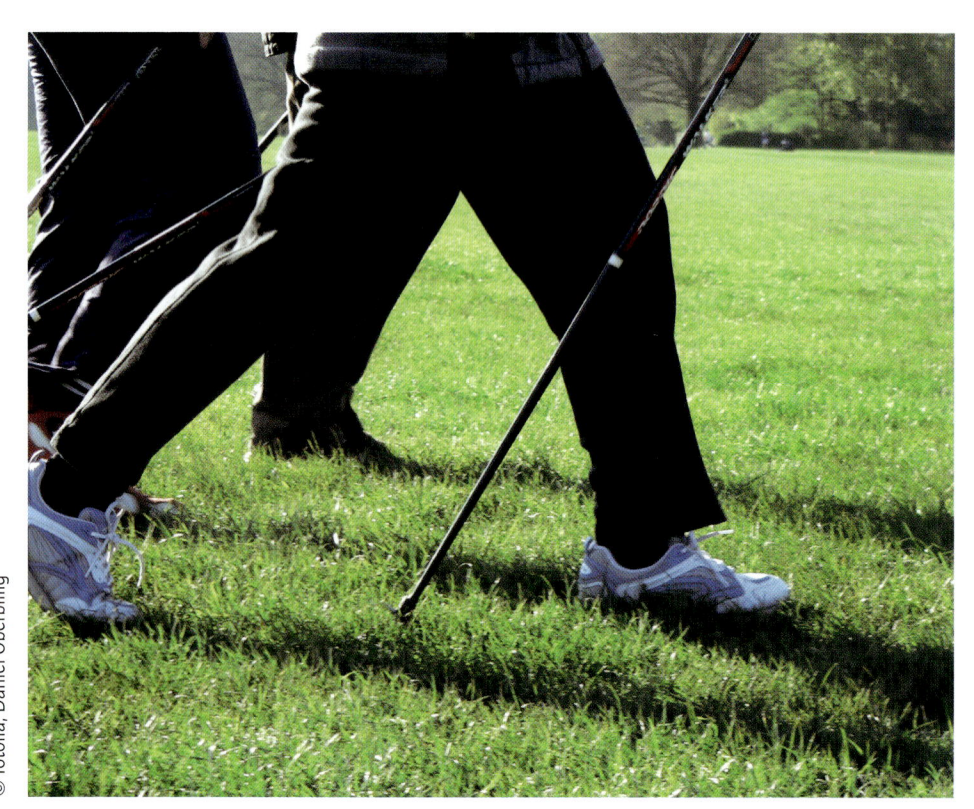

© fotolia, Daniel Oberbillig

STEP 2

Getting out and about and using your body in the outdoor environment is a great way to start stripping fat. The program below is based upon this. But if you have a little time, live in a wet environment or need to be close to home, then a treadmill can be used, using a similar approach to that provided below:

Time Objective: 30 minutes a day

Equipment
- Good quality walking shoes and socks
- Orthotics for people with flat feet (see a podiatrist)
- Comfortable sports clothing
- Water bottle
- Hat and sunscreen, especially if walking outdoors
- Mobile phone (in case of an emergency)

Choosing a Training Variable: Level 1 – 3

Training variables are designed to keep your body thinking. It's no longer just a 30-minute walk, it's a 30-minute challenge and it's fun. When starting out for the first few weeks, the aim is to keep things easy, starting with 10-minute intervals at normal walking pace to allow time for your body, its muscles, joints and energy systems to adapt and then gradually build this up to 20 then 30 minutes. Once you are able to walk easy normal walking pace (Level 1) continually for 30 minutes, the moderate (Level 2) and more challenging fast or hilly type regime (Level 3) can be introduced. With this in mind, always follow a challenging day (Level 3) with an easy one as this allows your body to recover appropriately. Taking a day off here and there is also fine but on these days I recommend getting a sports massage, reflexology or similar treatment to reward yourself for your efforts.

Below are a few examples of each category. Over time, with experience you will be able to design your own moderate and challenging routines.

Level 1: Easy Power Walk – Normal pace
- Walk at normal walking pace with good focus for 30 minutes on a flat or slightly undulating surface
- Taking the dog for a walk for 30 minutes
- Walk along the beach, around the park or other favourite area for 30 minutes or so

Level 2: Moderate Power Walk – Pick up the pace 10-30%
- Normal pace for 5 minutes; moderate pace for 5 minutes – repeated for 30 minutes
- 10 minutes normal pace; 10 minutes moderate pace (pick up the speed a little); 10 minutes normal pace
- 1 minute normal pace; 1 minute moderate pace – repeated for 30 minutes
- 30 minute walk around undulating area with a purpose for 30 minutes
- Forest walk for 30 minutes on established trail (with a friend)

Level 3: Challenging Power Walk – Pick up the pace 30-50% pumping the arms rapidly and walking with a purpose.
- 1 minute easy pace; 2 minutes fast pace (pump arms rapidly) x 10
- 2 minutes moderate pace, 1 minute fast pace (pumping arms rapidly); 1 minute easy pace; 8 kneeling push-ups – repeat this set six times changing exercises at each set
- 5 minute moderate pace; 10 x uphill walks for 1 minute with walk back down recovery (pump arms rapidly); 5 minute moderate pace recovery
- Forest walk in hilly terrain for 30 minutes or longer (with a friend)

Note:
- Similar principles can be applied to any cardiovascular exercise you decide to undertake as you become fitter. (i.e. treadmill, jogging)
- Each session you perform should be concluded with a period of stretching to maintain range of motion, muscle pliability and flexibility as well as drinking plenty of water.
- Always breath deeply when exercising, never hold your breath.
- Keeping a gauge on you pulse can help educate you about how hard you are working.

Power Walking Week – Sample

The best thing about the power walking plan is that you know you are going to exercise for 30 minutes, but the variables of intensity and the challenge is left up to you. This keeps exercise interesting and fun and coming back for more. WW is not just limited to power walking, you can include days where you cycle, swim, row or participate in an aerobics or dance class, pilates, water aerobics, boxing or any other aerobic activity you are interested – that's the flexibility of the WW program. If you do go to the gym, you can vary your exercises. For example, for a 30 minute workout, you could spend 10 minutes walking briskly on the treadmill, 10 minutes on the rowing machines and 10 minutes on the bike. Otherwise perform 30 minutes on one piece of cardio equipment and change the variables (speed and intensity) throughout.

The following table provides examples of how a week may be structured. As you progress, you will realize there are hundreds of variables you can apply. The key is always making them different and keeping the challenge on your body. In the first few weeks, gradually increase your time up to 30 minutes. Then as weeks roll by and you've got a routine, you can start to introduce other activities as shown below. There is plenty of flexibility, and plenty of choices you can make.

Week 1		Week 12	
Monday	Easy	Monday	Challenging
Tuesday	Moderate	Tuesday	Water Aerobics
Wednesday	Easy	Wednesday	Moderate
Thursday	Moderate	Thursday	Challenging
Friday	Easy	Friday	Easy
Saturday	Moderate	Saturday	Bike - Cycling
Sunday	Easy	Sunday	Moderate

Note: See Cardiovascular Exercise Variety chart on page 112 to address the type of activity you would like to perform

Establishing a Time to Exercise

With all the right ingredients now in place, in terms of Strength and Cardiovascular Training, one of the most important elements of exercising is establishing a time to fit it in. As you are introducing something important for your health and well-being, your lifestyle is about to change. One of the best times to exercise is first thing in the morning before breakfast. There are three main reasons; firstly, it's a very effective way for fat stripping. Secondly, you are more motivated and organized for the rest of the day. Third, if you are unable to perform it one morning, you have the rest of the day to fit it in. All things considered, anytime throughout the day you can exercise is fine – *morning, lunchtime, evening* – as long as you fit it in.

Just remember to exercise before eating, unless you have a condition that may require some form of food prior to exercising as per your doctors advice, or 1-2 hours after a meal when the food has digested. Along the way there will be a few small sacrifices you'll have to make, but that's normal because what you've done up until now hasn't worked and it's time for change. A shift in this direction is a positive one for your weight and your health. So, choose a time each day and stick with it. It might be four mornings a week, or one lunchtime and two afternoons. Look at your diary and your day and work out the most convenient time for you and make a commitment.

Monitoring your Progress

As your Personal Body Coach® I have put together a weekly planner that allows you to record and monitor your progress. It works like a 'checklist' each day with space available to cross off the activities once they're done. You can copy this planner each week and stick it up on the fridge or somewhere convenient. Otherwise write it into your daily diary so you have a 12-week record of what you've done. At the end of each week, you can assess how you did and make the appropriate adjustments. This way you become accountable to performing the exercises and achieving your goal. Refer to Step 3 for 12-Week Action Plan

WAISTLINE WORKOUT

Body Coach® Weekly Exercise Planner - Example

Exercise Objectives
- Upper Body Strength Training Routine (2-3 times a week)
- Lower (and mid) Body Strength Training Routine (1-2 times a week)
- Rate yourself out of 10 (1 poor; 10 excellent) for your strength training effort
- Planned Cardio Workout (i.e. Power Walking) – 30 minutes a day
- Tick the activity performed each day
- Record the actual time spent on each activity
- Success comes from accountability – so fill out planner out everyday
- Copy and place planner on fridge door or in diary
- Sample Planner Completed

(Sample planner completed, see page 128 for blank version for copying)

MONDAY

Strength Training
- [X] Upper Body
- [ ] Lower Body

Cardio Exercise
- [X] Easy
- [ ] Moderate
- [ ] Challenging

Time = 35 min
Training effort = 8 /10

Time = 20 min
Activity = Walk

TUESDAY

Strength Training
- [ ] Upper Body
- [X] Lower Body

Cardio Exercise
- [X] Easy
- [ ] Moderate
- [ ] Challenging

Time = 30 min
Training effort = 9/10

Time = 25 min
Activity = Walk

WEDNESDAY

Strength Training
- [X] Upper Body
- [ ] Lower Body

Cardio Exercise
- [ ] Easy
- [X] Moderate
- [ ] Challenging

Time = 38 min
Training effort = 9/10

Time = 30 min
Activity = Brisk

THURSDAY

Strength Training
- ☐ Upper Body
- ☐ Lower Body

Time = 0
Training effort = 0/10

Cardio Exercise
- ☐ Easy
- ☐ Moderate
- ☐ Challenging

Time = 30 min
Activity = Brisk/ Walk

FRIDAY

Strength Training
- ☐ Upper Body
- ☐ Lower Body

Time = 0
Training effort = 0 /10

Cardio Exercise
- ☐ Easy
- ☒ Moderate
- ☐ Challenging

Time = 25 min
Activity = Light/ Jog

SATURDAY

Strength Training
- ☒ Upper Body
- ☐ Lower Body

Time = 35 min
Training effort = 10/10

Cardio Exercise
- ☐ Easy
- ☐ Moderate
- ☒ Challenging

Time = 30 min
Activity = Boxing

SUNDAY

Strength Training
- ☐ Upper Body
- ☒ Lower Body

Time = 30 min
Training effort = 8/10

Cardio Exercise
- ☐ Easy
- ☒ Moderate
- ☐ Challenging

Time = 30 min
Activity = Brisk/Walk

Step 3
Successful Lifestyle Planning and Motivation

In this step you'll find the action plan in putting the Waistline Workout (WW) together incorporating the 12-Week Action Plan

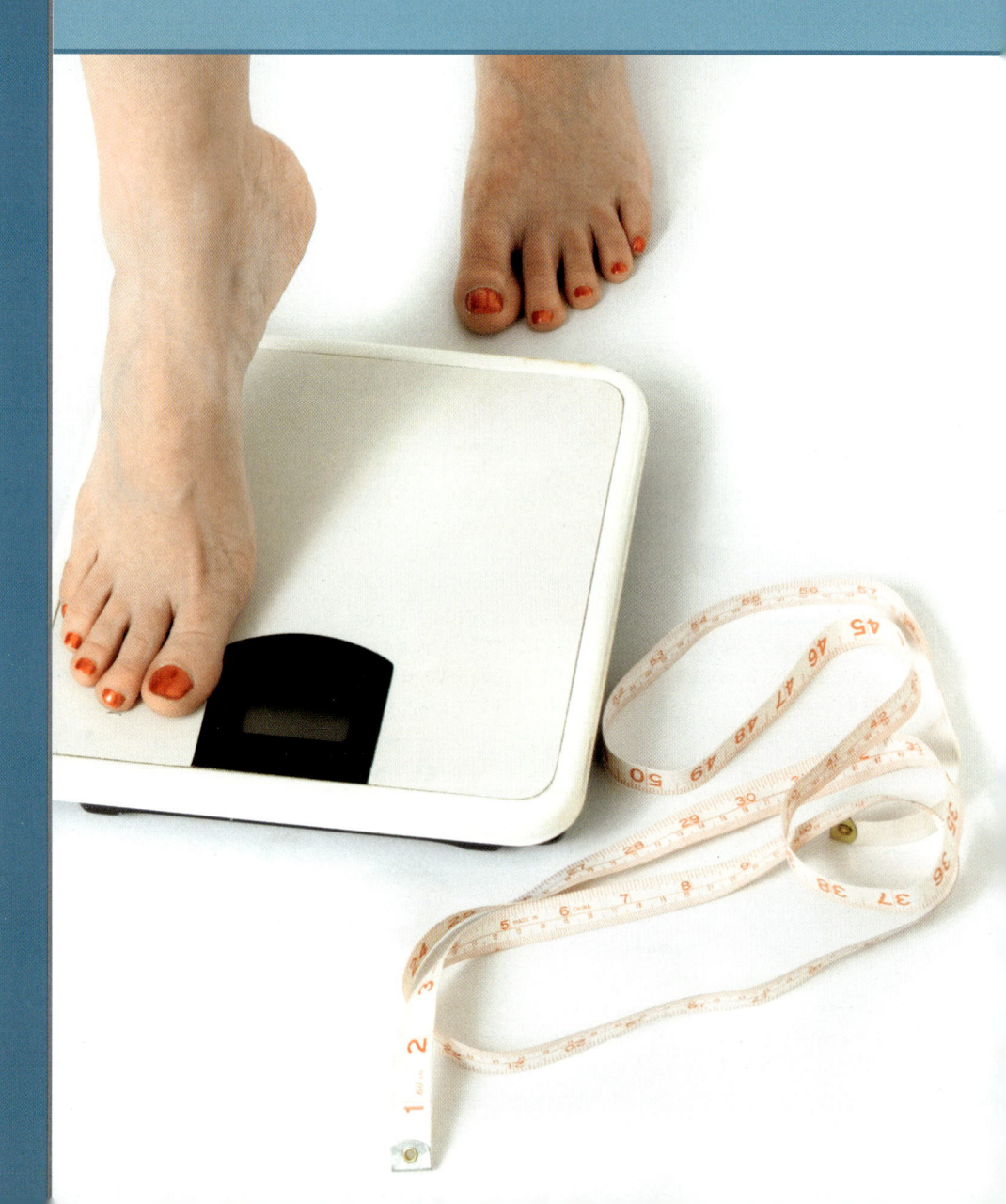

Accountability to Yourself – The Formula

Charting your progress is important because it keeps your focus on yourself and the tasks at hand. More importantly, it teaches you about being accountable and the role it plays in your success. On a building site, for instance, you are accountable to the project manager, who ensures the structure of the building is progressing successfully. In WW, various systems have been established that allow you to be accountable to yourself. Putting the information you learn from this book into practice is possible by being accountable to three important systems:

1. Body Coach® Daily Food Portion Chart
2. Body Coach® Weekly Exercise Planner
3. Monitoring Health Benchmarks as part of a Body Audit

Putting the Body Coach® Daily Food Portion Chart in practice each day with the guidance of the Recommended Dietary Intake (RDI), Portion Sizes and Menu Plans aims to keep you on track with your food intake. Meanwhile, the Body Coach® Weekly Exercise Planner is a summary chart that makes you accountable for the exercise you need to perform in terms of your strength and cardiovascular fitness each day. Using a diary to plan your exercise each day ensures it's booked, whereas the Exercise Planner itself allows you to record your daily effort.

The third important system you are accountable to is charting your progress of relative health benchmarks as part of the Body Audit. As you've learnt, long term weight loss success is a result of improving a number of lifestyle elements in terms of your diet, exercise, planning, habits, emotions, attitude, accountability and acceptance of the importance of living a healthy lifestyle.

Dealing with Habits and Emotions

In my experiences, some people who seem to eat well and exercise daily often do not achieve the body shape success they desire because there may be one small, but critical element that is holding them back. In many instances, this is often overlooked and they are unwilling to change (initially) because it is a habit that relates to an emotion or feeling or association that deals with stress. For instance, some people form relationships with chocolate, coffee, alcohol, cigarettes and other things that have become like a parent-child bond that is hard to break. It goes unnoticed for years because it has become part of their lifestyle routine and the feelings that they get when they consume it seems normal to them and why would they give it up?

The problem in weight loss arises because it contributes to elements such as excessive energy intake, insulin spikes or energy slumps or malnutrition. It's hard for some people to accept this is what's happening because it's been so normal for so long. Weight gain or bloating are a few indicators this is happening, because your health may have been tipped too far one way for too long. Getting in contact with your emotions, especially those related to seeking food or drinks (alcohol, coffee, soft drinks, etc.) for comfort or stress relief, need to be dealt with from the onset. It might take a while to accept and even turn this around because you've felt this way for a long while. However when you're ready to acknowledge it, positive changes will happen step-by-step. If this is a battle that you find is too hard to overcome by yourself, there are a number of health specialists who can help you in this instance, such as your doctor or psychologist.

In terms of food intake, it may just be that you are tipping towards one type of food too often such as consuming too many processed carbohydrates or fat. A balance between all food groups is essential for good health. By writing down what you consumed (food and drink) yesterday and so far today, provides a good indication of where you currently stand in terms of your eating habits when comparing these to the Recommended Dietary Intake and Body Coach® Daily Food Portion Chart. After writing these down and the time consumed, you can see your habits and the way you eat and drink each day. Remember, these are your normal habits because they have happened. Your goal is to turn these around. From this, questions you can ask yourself about your current habits include: (please tick those which currently relate to you)

- Do you skip breakfast, lunch or dinner?
- Do you eat too many treats (confectionary, cakes, cookies, etc.)?
- Do you eat a lot of foods high in fat (fast foods, chocolate, pastries)?
- Do you feel you lack planning of your meals?
- When stressed, do you seek comfort with food?
- Do you leave long gaps between meals, for example, longer than 3 hours?
- Do you drink less than 8 glasses of water per day?
- Do you feel you drink too much alcohol or soft drinks?
- Do you take too many coffee or cigarette breaks?
- Other: _____

If you answered yes to any of these questions, this can help you gauge where the scales are tipping and make the necessary changes in the right direction with the WW program at hand.

Positive Thinking

The mind is a very powerful tool. Positive thinking and healthy imagery help creative a positive environment for you to work with. With various food relationships and poor habits developing over one's lifetime, turning this around is controlled by the way you think. Positive thinking is a technique I use for helping athletes achieve optimal performance. It helps you come more in contact with yourself and the decisions you make by breaking negative barriers and becoming more focused on the task at hand.

To give you an example, below is a brief paragraph of positive thinking for achieving a healthy lifestyle and better body. Use this to create your own positive thinking passage that you can read to yourself out-loud (or your own version) each day in front of a mirror:

"Hello again! I'm looking at you because it's time to look after my health. The decisions I make today are positive ones that focus on my internal and external health and happiness. For me to achieve my long term goal, I need to eat well, drink more water and incorporate more exercise into my life – by focusing on what I should be eating – no excuses anymore. In the long term I will be rewarded with a much trimmer, slimmer, healthier and sexier body I am happy with. So, together lets make it happen! Yes – I can do it!

It's realistic to expect lapses or mistakes to arise from time to time. It's now about how you deal with these that matters. Use this above example as an inspiration for writing your own daily message and leading a healthy, positive, active and happy lifestyle. By making a commitment to WW and making your health a priority in your life, you will have much a clearer focus for achieving your goal. For more details visit: www.thebodycoach.com

Dealing with Emotional Bonds, Stress and Rut Eating

Rut eating refers to consuming the same food (drink or meals) over and over again, week-in and week-out at breakfast, lunch or dinner. To describe this further, if you eat the same breakfast everyday, this is rut eating. In simple terms, you are limiting the essential nutrient variety your body needs that can come with rotating meals at breakfast.

Over the years people often build an association with certain foods that become an emotional bond. The reason why I'm mentioning this now is because these rut eating and emotional patterns are often hard habits to break. Once something like this becomes part of your normal everyday routine, you may feel as though you are losing something if you give it up because it is seen as a comfort. This is important to understand because when people do start something new such as a new eating or exercise plan, if they don't stay focused and follow the plan they will more than likely go back to old ways with stressful days or when things get tough.

Dealing with stress is closely linked to rut eating, because when someone is stressed or emotional they generally find comfort from food, drinks (including coffee and alcohol), cigarettes and other forms. Various bonds build up over the years that need to be recognized first then modified. That's why being accountable to a Diet and Exercise Plan such as Waistline Workout is so important towards helping you break these bonds and build a new healthy lifestyle and reduce your waistline. I know this information may seem a little deep, but I believe that half of all diet failures are due to these speed bumps and lack of accountability. With the application of the Waistline Workout Diet and Exercise Plan, I have shortened these odds and made it much easier for you to achieve your goals. These plans allow you to be accountable to the program and keep you moving forward in the right direction.

By coming to terms with poor habits that may have formed, you will be able to experience a new outlook that brings with it a sense of confidence and motivation that helps you make the right decisions. This is because it matters to your health. Spend a few moments now to assess what habits you have built into your day as either rut eating or dealing with stress. Even ask your spouse, partner or friend and you will begin to understand this a little more. Below are a few example situations for you to refer to:

- Eating the same breakfast every day
- Drinking the same cup of coffee everyday, without fail at 9am
- Having cigarette breaks throughout the day
- Eating a chocolate bar every afternoon because you feel flat
- Eating 3 square meals each day

- Stopping off for a thick shake or donut everyday
- Drinking a glass or two of wine (or spirits) when you get home from work
- Food for comfort – chips or snacks in the evening after dinner
- Skipping breakfast, generally because you eat, drink or snack late into the evening
- Others....................

The thing is, even if you exercise regularly and eat well, various relationships formed with food and drinks are the final barricades stopping you from reaching your goal. Hence, if you've tried dieting in the past and failed, ask yourself why. Building new habits is therefore an important lifestyle change to make. If you reach a plateau in your weight loss, it's time to pinpoint these smaller elements because of the big part they play. There are a number of professionals (doctor, psychologist, hypnotherapist, etc.) that can provide further guidance. When you start eating well and exercising regularly, I can assure you these bonds will be the set of hurdles you will have to go over each day on your way to winning a WW Gold Medal. If and when you are ready to accept and work through these, great things will come in terms of weight loss and life in general. Most importantly, you'll be happier, healthier and slimmer around the hip, butt and thigh region.

Healthy Weight Range

From the healthy weight range chart for your height on page 56 record the healthy range (i.e. BMI Score between 20 to 25) and then complete the following equation to establish your weight loss goal.

Example calculation of goal weight:

- Sarah currently weighs 75 kilograms (165lbs) and is 1.63 meters tall.

- The healthy weight range for Sarah's height is: 53–66 kg (BMI Score between 20-25).

- Deduct current weight from BMI of 25. Example: 75kg – 66kg (BMI of 25) = 9kg.

- To calculate total body percentage to reach this point, divide the 9kg difference by current weight of 75kg and then multiply by 100 = 12% body weight loss required to fit within the BMI range.

- With proper nutrition and exercise weight loss of 0.5 to 1kg (or 1.1-2.2 lbs.) a week as well as smaller total body weight loss of 5% before reassessing is healthy, realistic and achievable. Weight loss beyond 5% total or any rapid weight loss requires monitoring by your doctor because major occurrences are happening within your body.

- In terms of reaching the initial BMI goal of being below 25, apply the 0.5–1kg weight loss per week principle. For Sarah, this equates to a period of 9–18 weeks to realistically reach this initial health goal.

- With this in mind you can see that weight loss only matters later in the equation. This way you can focus on the smaller details behind improving your health, fitness and diet for this long term goal to occur.

Complete the following to calculate your weight loss goal:

- Your initial starting weight in kilograms (or pounds) = _____ kg/lbs.

- List the health weight range for your height: _____ to _____ (see page 56).

- Deduct how many kilograms (or pounds) you are away from the higher BMI score of 25 from the healthy weight range: Your weight _____ kg/lbs. − _____ BMI of 25 in kilograms (or pounds) = _____ kg/lbs.

- Using 0.5 to 1kg (or 1.1-2.2 lbs.) weight loss per week, this equates to how many weeks to achieve this goal: ____ to ____ weeks

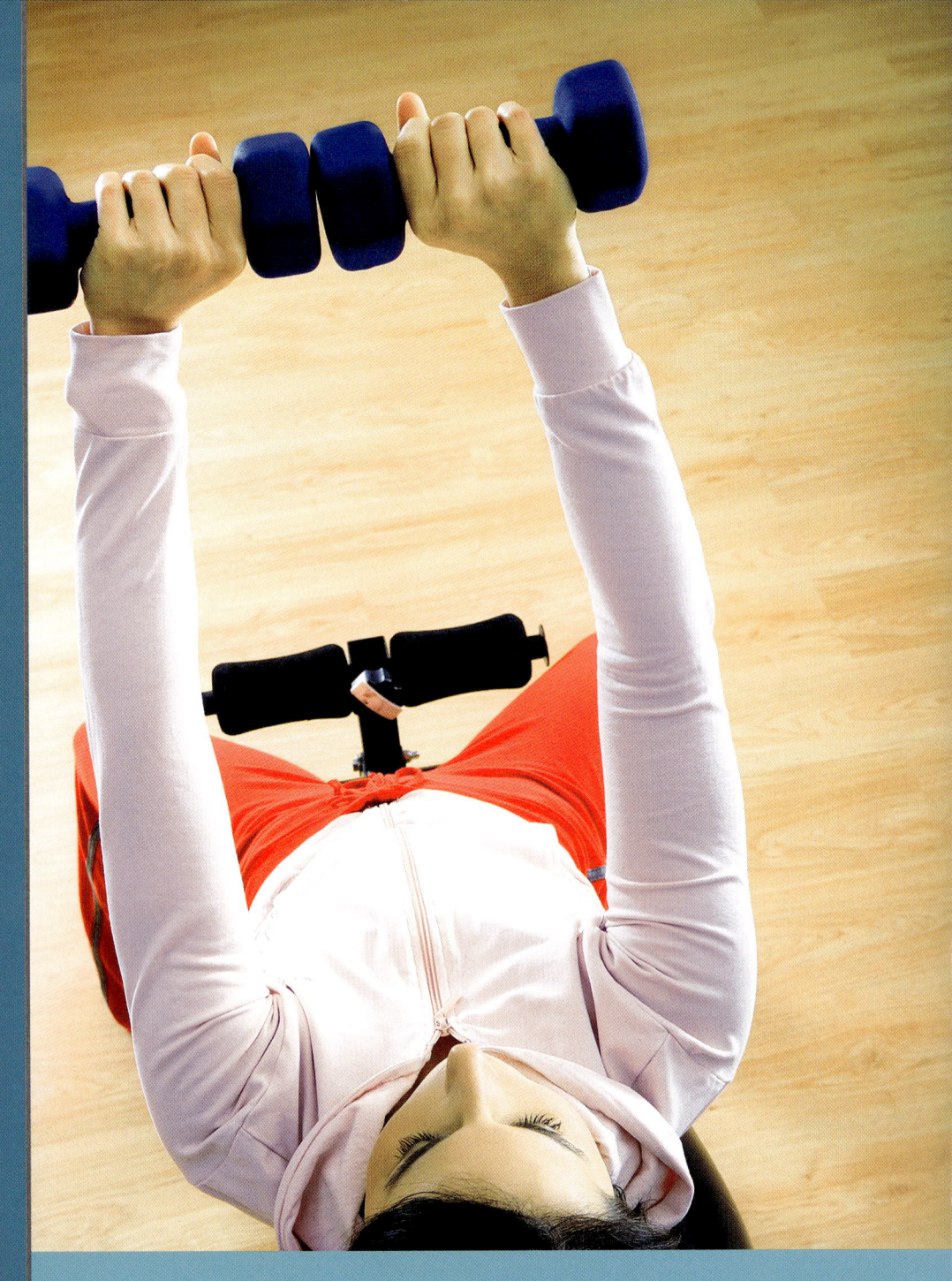

12-Week Action Plan

Putting it all into Practice

Use the following pages to implement and manage your program over the next 12 weeks. Refer back to steps within the book for guidance for each chart. Copy each page the desired amount of times required and keep in a diary or folder for daily use.

STEP 3

Week – _ of 12

- Copy this page to record your eating (every day of week).
- Utilize RDI tables in Step 1 to formulate and manage your daily eating plan.
- Plan and prepare your meals ahead of time and record your actual food portions consumed in table below.

Day (circle): M T W T F S S   Date: ____/____/_____

Body Coach® Daily Food Portion Chart

Complex Carbohydrates (Fiber)	Food Portions				Extra foods – for active people			
Cereals & Grains	1	2	3	4	5	6	7	8
Vegetables & Salads	1	2	3	4	5	6	7	8
Fruit			1	2	3			
Protein								
Animal (A)			1	2	3			
Plant (P)				1	2			
Calcium (C)			1	2	3			
Fat								
1 tablespoon of oil or margarine				1				
For every protein (A or P) source shade in one box	1	2	3					
Water (250ml Glasses)	1	2	3	4				
	5	6	7	8	9	10	11	12

Record any additional foods (or drinks) consumed below:

Note: Use this information to gauge your habits and making healthier food choices. Always work with your doctor to ensure the right eating plan for you. If you find yourself consuming an excess of only one or two types of food, you are limiting essential nutrients and you will need to shift your eating patterns to a more balanced approach that focuses on achieving all the RDIs.

Body Coach® Weekly Exercise Planner

Exercise Objectives
- Upper Body Strength Training Routine (2-3 times a week)
- Lower (and mid) Body Strength Training Routine (1-2 times a week)
- Rate yourself out of 10 (1 poor; 10 excellent) for your strength training effort
- Planned Cardio Workout (i.e. Power Walking) – 30 minutes a day.
- Tick the activity performed each day.
- Record the actual time spent on each activity.
- Success comes from accountability – so fill out planner out everyday.
- Copy and place planner on fridge door or in diary.

Week -   of 12   Weekly Starting Date: ____/____/_____

MONDAY

Strength Training
☐ Upper Body
☐ Lower Body

Time =
Training effort =   /10

Cardio Exercise
☐ Easy
☐ Moderate
☐ Challenging

Time =
Activity =

TUESDAY

Strength Training
☐ Upper Body
☐ Lower Body

Time =
Training effort =   /10

Cardio Exercise
☐ Easy
☐ Moderate
☐ Challenging

Time =
Activity =

WEDNESDAY

Strength Training
☐ Upper Body
☐ Lower Body

Time =
Training effort =   /10

Cardio Exercise
☐ Easy
☐ Moderate
☐ Challenging

Time =
Activity =

STEP 3

THURSDAY

Strength Training
☐ Upper Body
☐ Lower Body

Time =
Training effort =   /10

Cardio Exercise
☐ Easy
☐ Moderate
☐ Challenging

Time =
Activity =

FRIDAY

Strength Training
☐ Upper Body
☐ Lower Body

Time =
Training effort =   /10

Cardio Exercise
☐ Easy
☐ Moderate
☐ Challenging

Time =
Activity =

SATURDAY

Strength Training
☐ Upper Body
☐ Lower Body

Time =
Training effort =   /10

Cardio Exercise
☐ Easy
☐ Moderate
☐ Challenging

Time =
Activity =

SUNDAY

Strength Training
☐ Upper Body
☐ Lower Body

Time =
Training effort =   /10

Cardio Exercise
☐ Easy
☐ Moderate
☐ Challenging

Time =
Activity =

Weekly Training Notes: _____
_____
_____
_____

WAISTLINE WORKOUT

Monitoring Your Progress

The next element that plays an important role in the WW program is monitoring your progress. This keeps you updated, motivated and on the ball. Knowing your total body composition allows you to see changes that are occurring in centimeters coming off your body whilst your weight may stay the same with the body composition chart. To perform the measurements accurately apply the following:

- Record date of initial test, then every week afterwards for 12 weeks
- Measurements are taken in centimeters (cm) or millimeters (mm).
- Ask a family member or friend to measure you each week for consistency or simply do it yourself.
- Perform the measurements preferably at the same time for each test, for example, Monday at 9am.
- Total the sum of all measurements at the bottom of the table and compare each week to the first.

Weekly Body Composition Chart

Muscle	Location	1	2	3	4	5	6	7	8	9	10	11	12
1. Left Arm	Measure midpoint between elbow and shoulder												
2. Right Arm	Measure midpoint between elbow and shoulder												
3. Waistline	Measure around naval or belly button												
4. Hip	Measure around widest region of the hip and buttock												
5. Left Thigh	Measure the midpoint between the groin and knee												
6. Right Thigh	Measure the midpoint between the groin and knee												
7. Left Calf	Measure the widest region of the lower leg												
8. Right Calf	Measure the widest region of the lower leg												

Total sum of measurements in centimeters (cm) or millimeters (mm)

Blood Test Scores

A simple blood test can help determine your health status and provide clearer direction from your doctor on the correct pathway for you to follow. Visiting your doctor is also vital for gaining clearance to starting any new exercise program or eating plan. Ask the doctor for a blood test of the following areas as well as any other important element important towards improving your health. Always follow your doctors' recommendations.

Blood Test Scores	Preliminary Test Date:	1st follow up Date:	2nd follow up Date:
Cardiovascular (Cholesterol)			
Diabetes risk (Blood glucose)			
Anaemia (Haemoglobin)			
A liver function test (GGT)			
A kidney function test (Creatinine)			
Other test:			

WAISTLINE WORKOUT

WW Progress Summary Chart – Key Areas

The progress chart provides a specific summary of the major targets groups of the body, including the waistline and hip measurements, BMI score and weight in kilograms (pounds). It is used in addition to the body composition chart which enables you to see smaller transformations happening around your whole body. Transfer specific measurement from the body composition table to the progress summary chart below. Use this table and others to gauge your progress from week to week and where you first started from. To calculate your BMI score weigh yourself each week and perform the calculation on page 55.

Starting date:	Waist in cm or mm	Hip region in cm or mm	BMI Score (see page 55)	Weight in kg or lbs
Week 1				
Week 2				
Week 3				
Week 4				
Week 5				
Week 6				
Week 7				
Week 8				
Week 9				
Week 10				
Week 11				
Week 12				

Congratulations in completing your 12-Week Action Plan. Record the changes in your body form Week 1 to Week 12 and email this and your before and after photos to: thebodycoach@hotmail.com

Body Coach® Education and Products

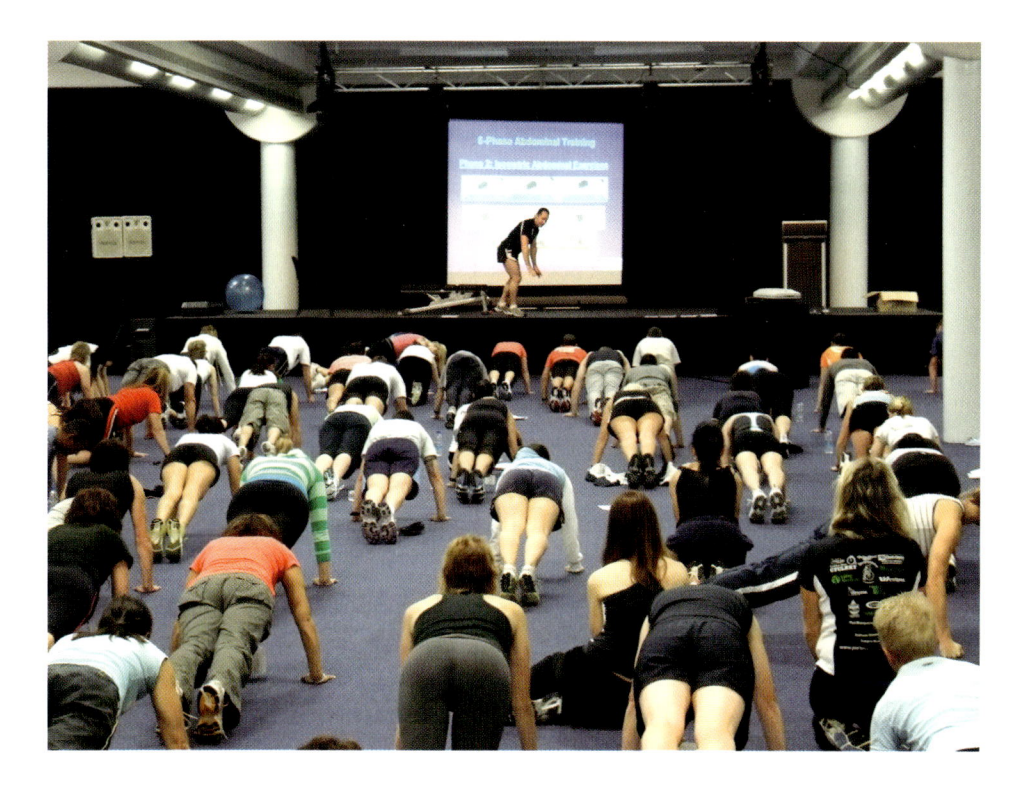

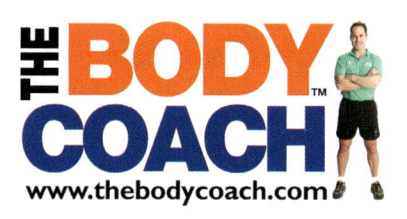

Paul Collins Presenting at International Fitness Conference, Sydney, Australia

Everything you need to know about fitness:
www.thebodycoach.com

Paul Collins
Speed for Sport

Speed is the number one factor linked to improving athletic performance in sport. Paul Collins' unique coaching guides you step-by-step through increasing speed for sport. The book offers over 100 of the latest speed training drills used by world class athletes and sporting teams for developing speed, agility, reaction and quickness.

208 pages, full-color print,
285 photos
Paperback, $6\frac{1}{2}$" x $9\frac{1}{4}$"
ISBN: 978-1-84126-261-1
$ 17.95 US / $ 32.95 AUS
£ 17.95 UK/€ 17.95

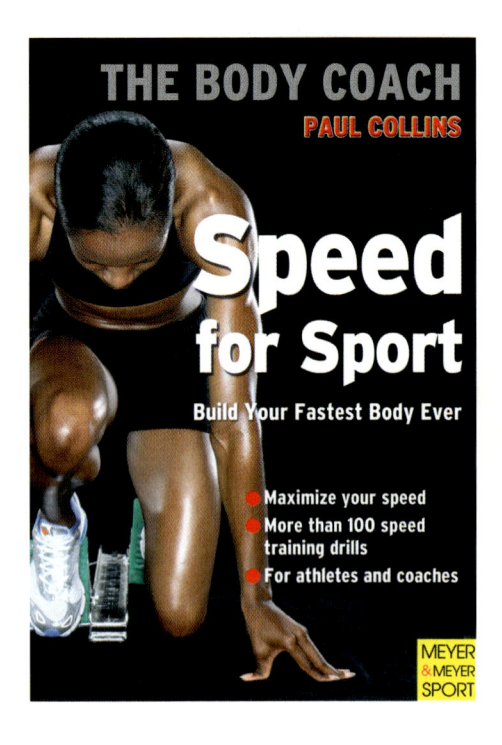

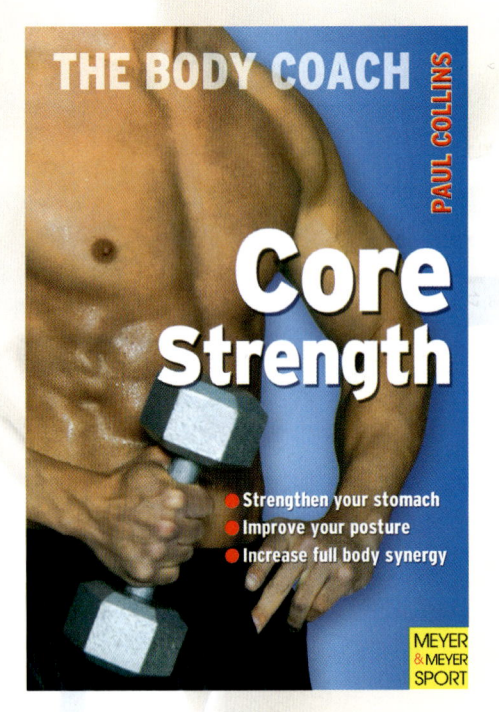

Paul Collins
Core Strength

Core Strength features practical, easy-to-follow exercises to help you build your strongest body ever using your own body weight. The Body Coach, Paul Collins, provides step-by-step coaching with detailed descriptions of over 100 exercises. As a substitute for lifting heavy weights, *Core Strength* provides body weight exercises for strengthening, toning and re-shaping every major muscle group in the body and staying in shape all year round.

200 pages, full-color print
200 color photos
Paperback, $6\frac{1}{2}$" x $9\frac{1}{4}$"
ISBN: 978-1-84126-249-9
$ 17.95 US / $ 32.95 AUS
£ 14.95 UK/€ 17.95

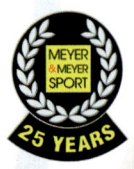

The Sports Publisher

Paul Collins
Strength Training for Women

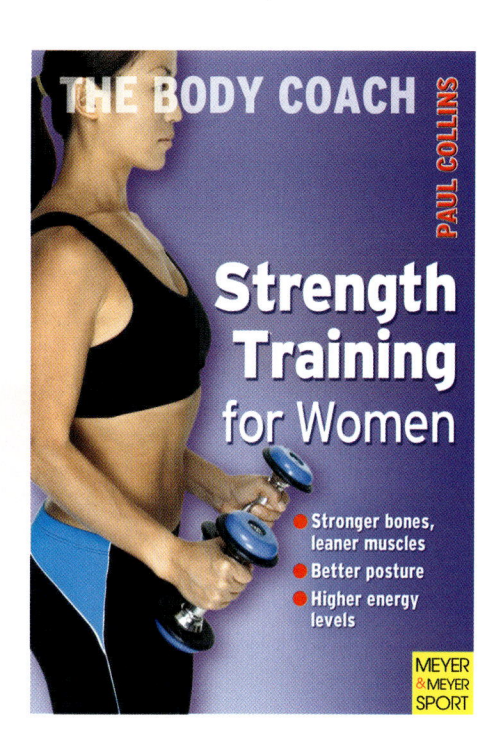

The combination of strength training, aerobic exercise and healthy eating habits has proven to be most effective for fat loss and muscle toning. *Strength Training for Women* has been developed as a training guide as more women begin to understand the health benefits of this activity. A series of strength training routines for use in the gym as well as a body weight workout routine that can be performed at home are included.

144 pages, full-color print
200 color photos
Paperback, $6^1/2$" x $9^1/4$"
ISBN: 978-1-84126-248-2
$ 14.95 US / $ 22.95 AUS
£ 9.95 UK/€ 14.95

Paul Collins
Functional Fitness

Functional Fitness features practical, easy-to-follow exercises for athletes, coaches and fitness enthusiasts in helping build your fittest body ever by simulating sports-specific and daily lifestyle movement patterns. The Body Coach®, Paul Collins, provides step-by-step coaching and workouts utilizing: body weight, fitness balls, medicine balls, plyometrics, resistance bands, stability training and speed training equipment.

144 pages, full-color print
332 photos, 9 illustr., 3 charts
Paperback, $6^1/2$" x $9^1/4$"
ISBN: 978-1-84126-260-4
$ 17.95 US / $ 29.95 AUS
£ 12.95 UK/€ 16.95

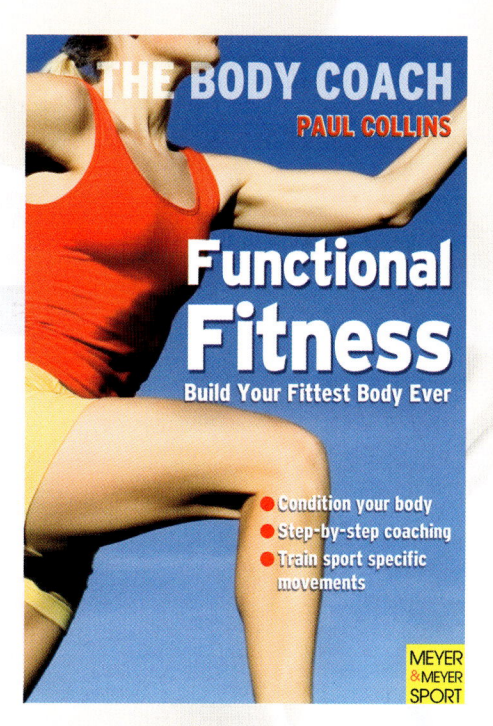

For more books from „The Body Coach"
visit www.m-m-sports.com

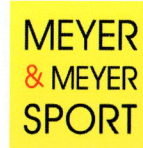

MEYER & MEYER Sport | www.m-m-sports.com
sales@m-m-sports.com

MEYER & MEYER SPORT

Photo & Illustration Credits:
Cover Photos: © fotolia/© fotolia, pixel
Cover Design: Sabine Groten
Photos: Paul Collins & Mark Donaldson